Coping with Prostate Cancer...

Prevention and Cure of Man's Most Common Cancer

by

Othniel Seiden, MD
& Jane L. Bilett, PhD

Proudly Published in the USA by

Boomer Book Series.com

ISBN: 1519438737

Dedicated to

The Prostate Cancer Foundation

CONTENTS

1

THE PROSTATE GLAND

Before we delve into understanding prostate cancer it will be very helpful to gain an understanding of what the normal prostate is, is like and how it functions normally.

The Normal Prostate Anatomy

The **prostate gland** is a small structure approximately the size and shape of a walnut. It is found just under the **urinary bladder**, in front of the **rectum** and behind the **pubic bone** of the **pelvis**. The **urethra**, the tube running from the base of the urinary bladder and down to and through the length of the **penis**, allowing both urine and semen to flow out of the body, travels directly through the prostate gland.

Two other important anatomic structures directly involved with prostate function are the **seminal vesicles** and **nerves** controling erection of the penis. The seminal vesicles are just above the prostate gland, two small glands that supply most of the fluid substance making up **semen** or male **ejaculate**. The nerves controlling erectile function are found running alongside and attached to the prostate gland. Because of this configuration and location of important anatomical structures around and through the prostate gland, treatment for prostate cancer can disrupt normal urinary, bowel, and sexual functioning despite best efforts by physicians or of treatment strategies.

Bands of muscle tissue, both at the base of the bladder and at the base of the prostate gland are known as the ***urinary sphincters***. These muscular valves normally remain tightly shut preventing urine stored in the bladder from leaking out before you are in a location convenient for evacuation. During urination, these sphincters are voluntarily relaxed and the urine can flow out of the bladder coursing the urethra and out through the penis. Some urinary incontinence or leakage will occur if the sphincter at the base of the bladder is damaged during prostatectomy or during radiation therapy.

Of considerable concern to many men and couples is the fear of surgical or radiation caused erectile dysfunction. If the erectile nerves are damaged during surgery or radiation, the ability to achieve an erection may be lost, however sexual desire is usually not affected. The loss of the prostate and the seminal vesicles through surgery or radiation renders men sterile. This would be similar to having a vasectomy.

2

PROSTATE SYMPTOMS AND THEIR MEANING
Urinary Obstruction...

A weak urinary stream or hesitancy in starting urination, or the need to strain to get urine to flow are symptoms of urinary obstruction. Also an intermittent urinary stream, one that starts and stops several times during a given urination is also a sign of urinary obstruction.? Dribbling or having difficulty in stopping urination, with excessive dripping at the end of flow is another symptom of urinary obstruction. There is often the sense of not being able to completely empty the bladder or worse, not being able to urinate at all. There can be several causes of urinary obstruction other than cancer. Most common of these benign causes is ***Benign Prostatic Hyperplasia*** or ***Hypertrophy*** otherwise known as ***BPH***

Benign Prostatic Hyperplasia (BPH)

Unfortunately most men will suffer some degree of BPH once they reach middle age or older. About the age that most women arrive at menopause most men will start to develop this benign swelling of their prostate gland. BPH is a factor in 20 percent of men by their fifties, 60 percent of men by the time they are in their sixties, and by the time they are in their seventies 70 percent of men have this affliction. Between 350,000 to 400,000 men a year in the United States will require some form of treatment to relieve their urinary obstruction caused by BPH.

Fortunately today, this treatment offers options not available before the past two decades. Until the 1990s, surgery was the primary treatment and radiation was coming into its prime. Today there is quite effective medical treatment for this disorder. Today most men are given a trial of medication before surgery is considered and in many cases this medical treatment remains adequate to control the problem of obstruction. Among men BPH is one of the most common diseases requiring treatment of one type or another as after age of sixty the majority of men will either be taking medication for BPH. However, BPH is still a fairly common cause of prostate surgery in men over the age of fifty-five.

It should be noted and emphasized that having BPH ***does NOT*** mean a man is more or less likely to get prostate cancer. BPH is not cancer and is in no way related physically or structurally to cancer. They're two vary different diseases. Furthermore, they involve different parts of the prostate gland. Prostate cancer generally originates in the outer or peripheral area of the prostate, growing outward and invading surrounding tissues. On the other hand, BPH originates from the inner zone of the prostate gland called the ***transition zone***, which is a ring of tissue around the urethra. Thus, in case of BPH, the growth is inward from the prostate's core, constantly tightening around the urethra obstructing the natural and free-flow of urination.

This leads to a differential diagnosis between BPH and Prostate cancer; BPH produces painful, annoying and difficult-to-ignore symptoms, while prostate cancer more often produces no symptoms for months or even years. That is why it is extremely imoortant for men to get yearly screening for prostate cancer; waiting for symptoms to show may make it too late for curative treatment.

What are the causes of BPH?

BPH seems to come with aging for reasons unknown. We do know that BPH involves two different types of tissue: glandular cells that make the prostate's secretions and smooth muscle cells, which contract to squeeze and expel those secretions into the urethra. In BPH the glandular cells start to build up and the smooth muscle tissue reacts to this buildup by tightening around the urethra, causing a biological damning up of the urine trying to escape the bladder through the urethra. It may be that the aging prostate simply becomes more sensitive to testosterone encouraging this benign growth.

Does BPH Run in Some Families?

Several studies have suggested that BPH does seem to run in some families, though this may be in less than 10% of all cases. In these few cases age doesn't appear to be the only major risk factor. A few men seem to have inherited genes that make them more prone to BPH than the general population. Understanding how this genetic influence works and specifically identifying the genes involved may soon provide major insight into the cause and cure of BPH and may one day help us prevent the disease.

The Major Problems BPH Can Cause.

The signs and symptoms of BPH vary from patient to patient. As the cell growth of Benign Prostatic Hyperplasia progresses, tissues become lumpy and bulbous nodules begin to form into characteristic clusters, or lobes. These lobes then tend to arrange themselves in one of three common configurations. There are *lateral lobe enlargements* that sandwich the urethra between them. As a man urinates, these lateral lobes can swing open and shut like double swinging doors, so despite their size, they may not produce much urinary retention or obstruction.

Another type BPH is *middle lobe enlargement*, where the lobes form around the bladder neck, plugging it causing great difficulty with urination. This form of BPH is difficult to ignore and men who have it are invariably more likely to seek medical treatment for relief for their symptoms. This type enlargement can happen in the bladder neck as well as in the urethra causing severe obstruction and other problems.

As the enlarging prostate gland squeezes in on the urethra, it tends to damn up or impede urine flow. This will usually manifest itself as *frequent* and incomplete urination, needing to go to the bathroom several times an hour. Frequently it causes *hesitancy*, having to wait uncomfortably for the urinary stream to start. Perhaps the most troubling symptom is *urgency*, the sudden sensation of needing to urinate, often culminating in involuntary urine leakage before reaching the bathroom. Among the common complaints of BPH patients is repeatedly awakening in the night to urinate; starting and stopping during urination with a constant feeling of fullness in the bladder. The classic summarizing symptoms of BPH thus are *frequency, urgency, hesitancy, disuria,* or painful urination. BPH may also lead to frequent urinary tract infections and can cause infection and/or damage to the bladder or kidneys. The longer urine is retained in the bladder the higher its chances are of it becoming a breeding pool for infection. If the bladder is never completely emptied it will more than likely have to be treated.

Even if the BPH causes less narrowing than needed to cause overt or obvious obstruction, thus causing few if any symptoms, the powerful bladder muscle may compensate for the narrowed urethra, with more intense contractions to force urine through. Over time, this extra effort can make the bladder less efficient. Eventually the bladder wall thickens losing much of its elasticity becoming unstable and over reactive. This can cause frequency, urgency, often-spontaneous loss of urinary control and dribbling. *Nocturia,* or the need to urinate often during the night is one of the most frequent complaints of BPH patients and their bed partners, making a good night's sleep impossible. If a BPH patient is unable to empty his bladder completely nocturia can become even worse.

Diagnosing BPH

Several other conditions can mimic BPH, so your physician will probably begin with a detailed medical history and a physical examination. Even if you have what seems a classic case of BPH it is still important for your doctor to know your entire medical history. Among the medical problems that may mimic BPH is injury to the urethra due to either external or internal trauma. These can cause a urethral stricture or scar tissue that narrows the urethra. Blood in the urine or bladder or penis pain might indicate a *bladder tumor*, or *stones* developed *in the kidney, bladder, or prostate*.

Prostatitis is another mimic of BPH. Prostatitis is a painful condition causing an inflamed, swollen, and tender prostate usually caused by a bacterial infection. The major complaint in prostatitis is pain in the *perineum*, the area between the rectum and the testicles and or aches, pain in the joints or muscles and lower back. Blood in the urine, *hematuria,* pain or burning during urination, *disuria,* and painful ejaculation may also be classic signs of prostatitis. Like BPH prostatitis is a benign ailment and it does not lead to cancer. Prostatitis is the most common cause of urinary tract infections in men Half of all men will probably experience some of these symptoms during their lifetime.

Bladder cancer, prostate cancer, and *neurogenic bladder* can also be produced BPH symptoms. Neurogenic bladder leads to trouble with bladder function caused by a neurological problem, such as Parkinson's disease or other interruption of normal nerve signals to the bladder muscle.

During your examination you will probably be asked to score the severity of your symptoms or how much they bother you on a questionnaire called the *International Prostate Symptom Score* (IPSS).

INTERNATIONAL PROSTATE SYMPTOM SCORE (IPSS)

0:   Not at all
1:   Less than 1 time in 5
2:   Less than half the time
3:   About half the time
4:   More than half the time
5:   Almost always

1. Incomplete emptying   0 1 2 3 4 5
Over the past month, how often have you had a sensation of not emptying your bladder completely after you finished urinating?

2. Frequency   0 1 2 3 4 5
Over the past month, how often have you had to urinate again less than two hours after you finished urinating?

3. Intermittency   0 1 2 3 4 5
Over the past month, how often have you found you stopped and started again several times when you urinated?

4. Urgency   0 1 2 3 4 5
Over the past month, how often have you found it difficult to postpone urination?

5. Weak stream   **0 1 2 3 4 5**
Over the past month, how often have you had a weak urinary stream?

6. Straining   **0 1 2 3 4 5**
Over the past month, how often have you had to push or strain to begin urination?

7. Nocturia   **0 1 2 3 4 5**
Over the past month, how many times did you typically get up to urinate between the time you went to bed and got up in the morning?

Total IPSS Score _____

Quality of life Score by Urinary Symptoms
How would you feel if you had to spend the rest or your life with your urinary condition just is it is now?

0: Delighted
1: Mostly Pleased
2: Satisfied
3: Equally Satisfied and Dissatisfied
4: Dissatisfied
5: Unhappy
6: Terrible

If your total score is:
0 to 7 Your symptoms are mild
8 to 19 Your symptoms are moderate
20 to 35 Your symptoms are severe

BPH is not a life threatening disease so all of its treatments are basically directed at symptom relief The main question you need to decide is whether you want to live with the symptoms your BPH is causing. These symptoms may increase in intensity and your lifestyle may also change. Thus, many men may choose to delay treatment. This is an individual decision that only you the patient can make.

Since BPH affects mainly the innermost core of the prostate, digital assessment of the gland through rectal examination may not disclose any enlargement at all. Therefore your doctor may employ other examination methods and tests to help make a diagnosis.

Ultrasound is an imaging technique that shows the shape and size of the Prostate Gland in a painless non-invasive manor. It creates an image by bouncing high-frequency sound waves off of the prostate tissue. There are two main methods used to perform the ultrasound, either through the abdomen, or transrectally using a wand inserted in the rectum. Beside determining the size and shape of the prostate gland, ultrasound may be helpful in showing other problems such as obstruction from kidney or bladder stones, or tumors or in determining how well the bladder is emptying.

Uroflowmetry is a method that measures the speed of your urinary stream and the amount of urine you pass, and is done as you urinate into an electronic measuring device.

Residual Urine Measurement or **Cyctometrics** can show if you're not emptying your bladder completely and will show how much residual urine you're leaving behind. This can be done indirectly by an ultrasound examination of the lower abdomen immediately after you urinate or directly by inserting a catheter into the bladder and measuring the retained urine. Excessive urinary retention may lead to chronic urinary tract infection or damage to your kidneys and will increase your urinary frequency and urgency. Cystometry is also a way to measure bladder pressure and contractibility if there is a question that the primary problem may be with the bladder rather than with the prostate. Cyctometrics are performed by threading a catheter through the urethra, and into the bladder allowing the monitoring of pressure changes as the bladder is filled with water.

Cystoscopy is a test usually performed in an outpatient setting. It is rather uncomfortable but not painful as topical anesthetics are usually applied into the urethra. Cystoscopy is most often used to assess the physical situation before an invasive procedure such as surgery is preformed. The *cystoscope* used in this procedure is a slender, lighted tube that is inserted into the tip of the anesthetized penis then slid through the urethra into the bladder. This allows the urologist to see the bladder, prostate, and urethra and spot anything abnormalities such as a stone, stricture, or enlargement. Furthermore, cystoscopy may also be used to rule out other conditions, such as the presence of bladder stones or bladder tumors.

Treating BPH

When BPH is first detected it may have few if any symptoms, perhaps having been picked up during a routine physical and rectal exam. For such a patient the first option may be watchful waiting. Men with mild symptoms who feel they can live with their symptoms for the time being. These minimal symptoms may stay the same, even improve, or they will probably with time get worse.

For men who display only moderate symptoms, the initial treatment considered should be trial of medical intervention. Medical treatment offers several approaches. One class of drugs frequently used is called *alpha-blockers*. There are two types of tissues involved in BPH; one is glandular, made up of cells that secrete the prostate's fluids while the other is smooth muscle tissue that contract and squeeze this fluid into the urethra. In BPH the glandular tissue enlarges and narrows the urethra and the smooth muscle tissue tightens around it narrowing the urethra even more. Alpha-blockers can counteract this by causing this muscle tissue to relax. These drugs are especially helpful in men with small prostates and moderate symptoms.

For men who on the other hand have significantly enlarged prostates, another class of drugs called *5-alpha reductase inhibitors* are often helpful in markedly shrinking the prostate gland. These drugs block the chemical that changes *testosterone* into *dihydrotestosterone (DHT)*, the form of male hormone found within the prostate gland. Physicians today have two drugs to combat this BPH problem, *Avodart (dutasteride)* and

Proscar (finasteride). Both block the activity of DHT. They appear to work equally well in shrinking the prostate's glandular tissue thus decreasing obstructive symptoms. These drugs may also slow or completely halt the progression of BPH. It must be pointed out that the relief of BPH symptoms lasts only as long as these drugs continue to be taken.

The use of both 5-alpha reductase inhibitors and alpha-blockers together have proven to work better together for some men. Men taking both drugs simultaneously seem to have a lower risk of developing acute urinary retention and were less likely to need invasive therapy. It should be pointed out that there is some concern that long-term use of 5-alpha reductase inhibitors may by artificially lowering PSA levels delay the diagnosis of prostate cancer.

Surgical Options

For those men with severe symptoms who do not respond to medical therapy, there are several effective surgical options. The gold standard of all surgical procedures for BPH is the *transurethral resection of the prostate TUR or TURP.* The TUR is performed under anesthesia, either general or spinal anesthesia. TURP is a surgical procedure, but the abdomen is rarely incised or opened. Only in vary rare cases in men with very large prostates does it become necessary to perform an open surgical procedure.

In a TUR, surgeons reach the prostate via the urethra by placing an instrument, a *resectoscope,* similar to a cystoscope through the penis. This instrument allows surgeons to view the prostate as they chip away at excess tissue. With today's modern technology the prostate's core is removed in fragments by means of electrosurgical cautery or laser. Because the resectoscope is slipped through the urethra, no skin incision is needed.

In recent years, several promising new techniques have been developed for the treatment of BPH. They all utilize a form of energy such as heat, radio waves, ultrasound, microwaves, and lasers to destroy cells that cause obstruction to the normal flow of urine through the urethra. These energy waves are aimed and focused then fired at the overgrowth of BPH tissue.

3

Risk Factors For Prostate Cancer

Most people are surprised to discover that prostate cancer is the most common non-skin cancer in America. Prostate cancer will affect 1 in 6 men. As men age the more likely you are to be diagnosed with prostate cancer. Although only about 1 in 10,000 men under the age of 40 will be diagnosed with prostate cancer, the rate shoots up to 1 in 15 men for ages 60 to 69. More than 65% of all prostate cancers are diagnosed in men over the age of 65. However, age is not the only risk factor for this disease; race and family history are important factors as well. African American men are 61% more likely to develop prostate cancer than Caucasian men and are shockingly nearly 2.5 times as likely to die from the disease. Men with a father, brother or son with a history of prostate cancer are twice as likely to develop the disease, while those with two or more relatives are nearly four times as likely to be diagnosed with the disease. The risk appears to be highest if the affected family members were diagnosed at a young age, the highest risk being in men whose family members were diagnosed before the age of 60.

These fact tend to point to genetic factors playing a role in why one man might be at higher risk, social and environmental factors, particularly **diet** and **lifestyle**, have a deciding effect as well. Recent research in fact has shown that diet modification might actually significantly decrease your chances of developing prostate cancer and markedly reduce the recurrence of prostate cancer. Diet and lifestyle can also help slow the progression of the disease. The significance of diet and lifestyle in regard to prostate cancer cannot be ignored.

Myths About
Prostate Cancer

Important as it is to understand the risk factors concerning prostate cancer, one should also know there are many myths having no link to this disease. Probably the most consistent myth or misconception is that having non-cancerous conditions of the prostate increase the risk of developing prostate cancer. *NOT true!* Granted, these non-cancerous conditions may cause symptoms not unlike those of prostate cancer and deserve full evaluated by a physician. However, there is no evidence that having BPH or prostatitis increases the risk for developing prostate cancer. Numerous research studies have shown the presence of BPH *does not* make a man any more or less likely to develop prostate cancer. Rest assured the growth of the prostate in men with BPH is *unrelated* to prostate cancer.

Prostatitis is an infection in the prostate, and while it is the most common cause of urinary tract infection in men, it too is unrelated as a cause of prostate cancer. Most treatment strategies are designed to relieve the symptoms of prostatitis, which include fever, chills, burning during urination, or difficulty urinating. Again, numerous research projects have shown the presence of even frequent prostatitis does not make a man any more or less likely to develop prostate cancer.

Sexual Activity, and very frequent ejaculation have been rumored to increase prostate cancer risk. ***NOT true!*** Even at very high frequency, sexual activity has no link to prostate cancer. In actuality the good news is that studies have shown that men who reported more frequent sexual activity and ejaculations had a lower risk of developing prostate cancer. Whoopee!

4

Prevention of Prostate Cancer... Nutrition

Ultimately the goal here is to prevent men from ever developing prostate cancer. Of course this lofty goal has not yet been achieved. However, much progress has been made in the past two decades. Numerous risk factors for prostate cancer, both genetic and environmental, have been identified and eventually more research will narrow the gap between our hopes and reality.

To date considerable progress has been made to delay the development and progression of prostate cancer. *Finasteride and dutasteride,* the drugs frequently used for treatment of BPH, have shown a potential function in slowing the development and progression of prostate cancer. Furthermore, research around diet and lifestyle changes has shown considerable success in reducing the risk of prostate cancer development as well as its progression. Slowed progression of the disease lets patients with prostate cancer live longer, fuller and more normal lives.

Nutrition & Prostate Cancer

The more researchers delve into the relationship between diet and prostate cancer it becomes clearer that nutrition has a dramatic effect on this disease. Diet and nutrition may have a greater effect on the development and progression of prostate cancer than on any other cancer afflicting humankind. This is a strong statement, but the growing body of research appears to bear this out with each passing study.

Of all the risk factors for prostate cancer afore mentioned, age, family history or genetics, race, lifestyle and nutrition, only lifestyle and nutrition do we have any power to control. In the future with *DNA* and *Stem Cell* research we may get some control over genetics and race. But in this day and age our best hope for prevention and delay of this disease lies in nutrition and lifestyle. Our environment and our diet has a tremendous influence on the way our body functions and especially *dysfunctions*. This is not only in the case of prostate cancer, but nearly all the illnesses and diseases that afflict humans.

Prostate cancer research over the past decade has continuously shown with a dramatic growth of documentation, that ingesting certain nutrients you may well decrease your chances of developing prostate cancer. Furthermore, these same nutrients appear to reduce the likelihood of having a recurrence of prostate cancer and slow progression of the disease.

Protective Nutrition
Against Prostate Cancer

Fruits and Vegetables

Fruits and vegetables are a rich source of vitamins, minerals, and naturally occurring chemicals, which have strong cancer-fighting properties. The *US Department of Health and Human Services* as well as the *US Department of Agriculture* recommend that all of us should eat 5 to 9 servings a day of fruits and vegetables. In addition to the benefits that they bring in fighting prostate and other types of cancers, there is strong evidence that an increased consumption of fruits and vegetables may decrease our risk of heart disease, stroke and a growing variety of other illnesses, diseases and physical and mental disorders. Adding a wide variety of fruits and vegetables into your diet will help you achieve a healthier lifestyle.

Vitamins and Minerals

Vitamins and minerals found in foods and supplements play an important role in the body's many processes and functions. Those found in natural foods are in most cases more valuable and less expensive than those produced by man or woman. Many of these vitamins and minerals function by monitoring the balance between cell growth and cell death, particularly cancer cell growth and cancer cell death. Upset of this balance in growth and death of cancer cells may allow them to multiply and spread. Research over the years has shown clearly that the loss of a number of vitamins and minerals can contribute to cancer cell growth and conversely, increased vitamin and mineral nutrition either through foods or supplementation can slow the development and progression of cancers and other diseases.

Healthy vitamin and mineral rich foods

The following table of foods and supplements are of particularly value for prostate health:

Vitamin A- Apricots, lettuce, spinach, other green vegetables, livers

Vitamin B6- Fortified cereals, chickpeas, nuts, grains

Vitamin C- Citrus fruits and juices, red peppers, grape juice, potatoes

Vitamin D- Sunlight, fortified milk

Vitamin E- Fortified cereals, tomato-based products, nuts, spinach

Beta-carotene- Carrots, pumpkin, sweet potatoes, spinach

Calcium- Dairy products, collard greens, sardines with bones

Lycopene- Tomato-based products, watermelon, pink grapefruits, guava, papaya

Selenium- Nuts, fish, whole-grain wheat flour, garlic

Zinc- Raw or cooked oysters, beef, crab

Source: U.S. Department of Agriculture, Agricultural Research Service. 2004. USDA Nutrient Database for Standard Reference, Release 17. Available at:
http://www.nal.usda.gov/fnic/foodcomp/Data/SR17/wtrank /wt_rank.html.

There are both benefits and drawbacks to Supplementation

The mega doses in some supplement preparations can be harmful. Since we often tend to eat a wide variety of foods, many of which are packaged foods and fortified with additional vitamins and minerals, true vitamin and mineral deficiency is relatively uncommon in the United States. Therefore, some of our available supplement may actually become over-supplements. This can become a problem with certain vitamins, such as vitamins A, D, E, and K, which are not easily excreted by the body. If taken in excessivly high doses, they may build up in the body and actually cause damage to the body's systems and function. Therefore, before you explore the adding supplements to your diet to help delay prostate cancer or progression, or any other health problem, talk with your doctor or nutrition counselor about establishment of a safe balance of healthful vitamin or mineral supplementation.

Staying within the recommended ranges for vitamin and mineral intake is a smart choice

	Recommended Intake*	Upper Intake Level†
Vitamin A	3,000 IU/day	10,000 IU/day
Vitamin B	61.7 mg/day	100 mg/day
Vitamin C	90 mg/day	1,800 mg/day
Vitamin D	400 IU/day	2,000 IU/day
Vitamin E	22.5 IU/day	1,500 IU/day
Calcium	1,200 mg/day	2,500 mg/day
Selenium	55 mg/day	400 mg/day
Zinc	11 mg/day	40 mg/day

Values are for healthy males aged 19-70.
*Recommended dietary allowances or adequate intakes to be used as goals for individual intake. †The maximum level of daily nutrient intake that is likely to pose no risk of adverse effects; represents total intake from food, water, and supplements.
Source: Institute of Medicine of the National Academies. Dietary reference intakes. Available at (pdf file).
http://www.iom.edu/Object.File/Master/21/372/0.pdf

Use Dietary Fats and Red Meat in Moderation

Though red meat is an excellent source of protein, iron, zinc, vitamin B6, and vitamin B12, our common American diet usually is excessively high in red meat and animal fats and too low in fiber, fruits, and vegetables. This type of food ingestion has long been understood to be associated with high risks of obesity, heart disease, and numerous cancers, prostate cancer among them. Although the data are still preliminary, results to date suggest that dietary fats and red meat can negatively influence the growth of prostate cancer cells and therefore deserve attention. In addition to the suspected causative effects of meats and fats on cancer, preparation of these foods may also have a detrimental effect. One of the great culinary loves of most American is the barbecue grill. Unfortunately, the charring caused by this form of meat preparation been linked to a host of carcinogens or cancer-causing substances. ***Heterocyclic amines,*** a group of carcinogens identified first in the 1970s, were added this year by the U.S. Department of Health and Human Services to the list of substances reasonably anticipated to be human carcinogens. Heterocyclic amines are found in grilled beef, pork, chicken, lamb, and fish. Because carcinogens are often formed through direct contact with an open flame, it is questioned whether reducing the amount of charring over open flames or glowing embers can reduce the amount of heterocyclic amines.

Further research is being carried out to find out if heterocyclic amines are reduced in the body by increasing the eating of *cruciferous vegetables*, which have been shown to help reduce and eliminate carcinogens from the body. Brussels sprouts and broccoli appear especially able to help excrete these carcinogens form the body. When these vegetables were removed form the diet the levels of the carcinogens were again elevated. Findings to date seem to indicate that limiting the intake of red meat and fats might decrease the risk of developing prostate cancer.

It would probably be wise to try new methods for cooking lean red meat other than grilling, such as stewing, roasting, or even broiling, while also incorporating more fish into your diet. Dietary changes to eliminate charred and grilled meat would be an ideal goal though unlikely, so when you grill or barbecue, try to minimize the charring of the meat.

It is important to note that although cutting back on food intake and managing your portion sizes are very important for weight management strategies, when it comes to prostate cancer prevention, the *quality* of the food is often far more important than the *quantity* ingested. Instead of using an Alfredo sauce on your bowl of pasta, you exchange the high fat topping for a sauce with fresh tomatoes and sauce, broccoli florets, and small chunks of tuna This simple and easy exchange has added *lycopene*, *sulforaphane,* and *omega3 fatty acids*, all healthy carcinogen fighters to your meal. Discuss oter simple exchanges of healthy foods for unhealthy eating habits with you r physician or nutritional advisor. It is also advisable that you don't make too many radical changes at once. Gradual change lets you develop more lasting lifestyle and eating habits.

Important as dietary and lifestyle changes may be to retarding and preventing prostate cancer, be sure you discuss with your physician before making any nutritional changes in your dietary habits, especially if you have medical conditions that also affect your diet and lifestyle, such as diabetes, hypertension, elevated lipids, or heart disease.

Every small step toward a general healthier lifestyle is as well an important that will ultimately contribute to your efforts in battling this disease.

5

Prevention of Prostate Cancer... Exercise

When it comes to disease prevention and cure next to good nutrition for achieving general good health comes exercise. It is a fact that a healthy body is far more resistant to injury, illnesses, and chronic diseases. Further more obesity, which is epidemic in America, is due to both poor nutrition and lack of exercise; to remedy one without the other makes the job much more difficult in not impossible. Just as ingesting of excessive meats and fats ads to your risk factors for prostate cancer, so does excessive fat storage in your body.

If you are heavy and have been sedentary then your weight is probably due to an excess of fatty tissue. It's all that stored up energy you're saving up for that day you'll have to take action. Well now is the time to take action! Let's get moving and burn off that stored up energy by using it to build endurance, muscle tone and renewed strength. The time has come to rebuild yourself into as healthy a person as you have the potential to become.

Exercise physiologists have shown that to get maximum benefit from an aerobic exercise program you must maintain your ideal exercise pulse rate, to be discussed later, for 45 minutes and preferably for one hour. In addition to this you should do enough exercise to burn off at least 2,000 Calories a week exercising at least five and if possible seven days a week. Keeping these facts in mind, walking is the best, and in most cases, the only exercise to fill these requirements. There are very few, if any, other exercises most of us can keep up for 45 minutes, much less for a full hour, while maintaining our ideal exercise pulse rate. But by brisk walking most of us can accomplish just that. If you can't do it now, in most cases, you will be able to in just a few weeks of conditioning.

When you walk a mile on level ground and weigh around 150 pounds, regardless of the speed with which you do it, you will burn off about 100 Calories. That's because calories burned is a function of weight through distance regardless of the time it takes. If you are less than 150 pounds you'll burn a little less, if over 150 a little more. For once we heavyweights get a break; most of us will burn 150 to 200 calories an hour when we do that mile. Thus, if you walk four miles in one hour, you'll be burning off at least 400 Calories each day and in only five days will burn your 2,000 Calorie weekly quota. If you walk six or seven days that's all the better. And if you walk a full hour you'll be maintaining your ideal exercise pulse rate for over 45 minutes, even allowing for a warm up and cool down period. I can think of no other exercise that so perfectly meets all these physiological criteria for a good aerobic workout.

Now let's determine *YOUR IDEAL EXERCISE PULSE RATE.* Your personal rate is determined by your age. The formula is as follows:

220 minus your age times .70 **(220 - age)* .70**

Thus, if your age is 65 years old, your ideal exercise pulse rate would be:
220 - 65 = 155   155 X .70 = 108

So your ideal exercise pulse rate would be 108 beats per minute. In other words, you would want to walk at a speed that would maintain your pulse at 108 beats per minute for 45 minutes to one hour.
There are three other pulse rate figures you should know about; *your minimum exercise pulse rate ... your maximum exercise pulse rate and your resting pulse rate.*

Your minimum exercise pulse rate =
220 - your age X .60

Your maximum exercise pulse rate =
220 - your age X .80

Thus, if you are 65 years of age your minimum exercise pulse rate would be 155 X .60 = 93 beats per minute and your maximum exercise pulse rate would be 155 X .80 = 124 beats per minute.
What these figures mean to you is that if you are walking so slow that your pulse rate is less than your minimum exercise pulse rate, it is doing you little aerobic good. If you are walking so fast that your pulse is beating faster than your maximum exercise pulse rate, you should slow your pace enough to drop

below that number. If you are indeed 65 years of age you should try to walk fast enough to keep your pulse between 100 and 120 beats per minute for 45 minutes to an hour, preferably at 108 to 110 beats per minute.

Please note if you are taking a Bata Blocker or other medication which slows your pulse it may be difficult to reach the above levels and you should check with your physician to determine your ideal exercise levels.

Before we talk about resting pulse rate, find your minimum, maximum and *ideal exercise pulse rates* on the line with your age in the table below. Memorize them.

TABLE OF EXERCISE PULSE RATES (E.P.R.)

Age	Minimal EPR	Ideal EPR	Maximum EPF
20-30	114-120	133-140	152-160
30-40	108-114	125-133	144-152
40-50	102-108	119-125	136-144
50-55	90-102	115-119	132-136
55-60	96-99	112-115	128-132
60-65	93-96	108-112	124-128
65-70	90-93	105-108	120-124
70-75	87-90	101-105	116-120
75-80	84-87	98-101	112-116
80-85	81-84	94-98	108-112
85-90	78-81	91-94	104-108
90+	75	90	104

Resting Pulse Rate

A major problem of most heavy sedentary people is that their pulse has been doing too much resting. And surprisingly, by starting an exercise program your pulse will actually rest more. The importance of your resting pulse rate is that it is one of the best measures of your cardiovascular improvement as you progress in your walking program. As you get into better fatness your resting pulse will actually slow down, as will your exercise pulse rates. But resting pulse rate is the best way to measure this improvement. To determine your resting pulse rate, take it first thing upon awakening in the morning before you get out of bed. If you can't take it then, count it after sitting or lying down completely relaxed for about ten minutes. Try to take it at the same time and under the same conditions each day. As you get into better condition your resting pulse will become lower and lower. Other measures of your improvement have been discussed in chapter 1, *Better Ways To Measure.* Review it.

Now let's get back to your exercise goal ... to develop your cardiovascular/cardiopulmonary health so you can *walk an hour at your own ideal exercise pulse rate* ...and going on to achieving and maintaining your best fitness potential.

Decide with your physician what your beginning level of exercise should be. If in doubt, start out with a minimal walk. Do what you know you can do even if it is only a few steps. If you are really very obese and walking is a burden for you, start out in a swimming pool. Simply walk back and forth in the shallowest water that is comfortable for you. Walking in water supports the weight of your body taking the burden off your legs. Walk as far as you comfortably can and add a width each day. As your legs strengthen and endurance increased you will see that this endurance caries over to walking on dry land. Walking against the resistance of water is excellent exercise and will start to burn off the excess fat deposits and begin building and toning muscle.

Eventually transfer to walking on land, again starting out with a distance that is comfortable for you. If you do it with more ease than you expected, then add a few more steps with each walk you take. Even if you're just getting out of a sick bed and your walks are only a few feet, do them as often in the day as you can. Your walking program will progress at a much faster pace than you can imagine. Until you can walk for twenty minutes without a stop, don't feel you have to push yourself too far beyond comfort. The important thing is to make each walk a little further and/or a little faster than the last. And *walk every day.* Make it part of your daily routine, preferably at the same time each day. It has to be scheduled to give it its proper priority among all the other things you do each day. In fact it *has to be at the very top of your priorities.* Realize, *any day you don't find time to exercise walk, you're saying everything you do that day is more important than your_health!* Your *health is your most important asset!*

To help you measure your progress, record on paper how far you walk today and how long it takes you. At the end of each week compare and chart your progress. You'll be amazed at the rapid improvement. There are tables to record your progress at the end of this book.

When you finally get to the point where you can walk a full hour non-stop ... and it will happen sooner than you or your doctor think ... you should start to increase your pace a little each day until you reach your ideal exercise pulse rate. Once you reach that level it does not mean you won't improve any more. Your physical condition will still improve gradually and you'll know it because you'll have to walk faster over time to get you up to your ideal exercise level. Thus your ideal exercise pulse rate will become another measure of your continuing cardiopulmonary health development along with your resting pulse rate.

Let's review the other measures of your gains in physical health:

1. You will feel better all over with fewer aches and pains. When something does bother you you'll bounce back quicker. An active body becomes a supple stronger body and more resistant to injury.

2. You'll look better, have more muscle tone throughout your entire body. You may not lose much weight, but you'll have less fat and look trimmer. People will take notice of the change and will comment on your new physique.

3. You'll be happier, more confident, have more energy and interests. You'll break new frontiers of activity every day. And that increased activity will itself burn off more calories. Activity breeds on activity.

4. You'll sleep better, might even snore less.

5. You'll find your joints are more supple and limber and less subject to pain, injury and stiffness. Recent studies have shown that even people with arthritis in their hips and knees are improved with walking. Here again, walking in a pool might be a necessary first step.

6. You'll think better, clearer and more creatively because of the improved circulation to your brain. And as you become more active you will find more interesting challenges for your mind to replace those sitcoms that have been hypnotizing you on the tube and jellying your brain.

7. You'll want to get out and do things you thought you'd never be interested in again. More important, others will probably begin inviting you to join into their activities. The more active you are the more people you will meet and the better chance you have of making new friends with common interests.

8. You'll enjoy friends and relatives a lot more and they'll enjoy you. As your interests broaden and activities increase the more you'll have in common with friends and loved ones. You'll just be more fun to be with than a TV watching couch potato.

9. You'll stop feeling sorry for yourself and may well want to help others achieve your state of health and happiness for themselves. The

best way to maintain your lifestyle for life is to encourage others to the same healthy ways.

10. You'll start looking for and setting new goals for yourself. As you start to reach your first goals you'll realize that more lofty aspirations are also attainable. Once you get yourself off that couch the world has no limit.

11. You'll start thinking of your bright future instead of living in the past ... realizing that your life is still very much in front of you. A healthy person can expect to live an active productive and fun life well into nine or more decades.

12. Your sexual drive, prowess and pleasure should increase. A healthy person can expect to have an active sexuality throughout his/her entire life. And it's better when you have the energy, vitality and are trimmer, even if you don't lose any weight. Exercise can often eliminate sexual dysfunctions which are often due to poor physical condition.

So get up right now and take your first steps toward that new life ahead of you!

A lot has been written about stretching and warming up before you exercise. I don't even think it's a good idea for skinny folks. It's too easy to overstretch muscles that are cold causing injury. If you're heavy the danger is even greater. I feel the best warm up for walking is walking. Spend the first four or five minutes of your walk gradually working up to your best exercise pace. Start out at a comfortable walk and gradually increase your stride and speed until you fall into a brisk rhythm that is adequate to give you a good cardiovascular workout.

More important than the warm up to your walk is an adequate cool down period at the end of your walk. *Never, never* just stop after you've been walking at your ideal exercise pulse rate or faster without cooling down with a slower walk. Reduce your speed and continue to walk until your pulse is slowed to under your minimal exercise rate or less than 110, whichever is lower.

Then if you want to do some stretching exercises, do them after your workout when your muscles are warmed and more flexible. If you start your walk slow and easy and build up your pace, the muscles will warm up and limber safely. Then do your stretching after the vigorous workout. You will get all the benefits of stretching without the danger of injury. Furthermore, the post exercise stretching will keep you from getting stiff and painful muscles and joints after too vigorous a workout.

What about other sports? And what if you can't walk?

As for those few of you who can't walk due to a real physical handicap, the same principles apply. You must find an activity that will keep your pulse rate at its ideal exercise level for 45 minutes to an hour. Consider swimming, rowing or bicycling on a stationary rowing machine or bike or other water exercises such as pool aerobics. You may find that these exercises will improve your condition to where you will be able to work into a walking program after all.

For those of you confined to a wheel chair, 45 minutes to an hour of wheeling yourself around a park is an ideal workout. Begin the same as recommended for the walking program, an easy spin at first, gradually adding to your time and distance and then adding to your speed until your working at your ideal exercise pulse rate for 45 minutes to an hour. You may even become interested in other wheelchair sports or more competitive racing and marathons. Push your activity as far as you can.

If you are bedridden or otherwise confined by your physical health, ask your physician about a physical therapy consultation to determine your true potential and how to reach it. There are very few who can do no exercise, but for those few, you can still maximize your fitness and life span by following the other lifestyle changes recommended in this book.

As for other exercises and sports activities, they are great if you enjoy them, but they do not replace your walking program. You should participate in as many exercise or athletic activities as you enjoy, over and above your walking program. If you are heavy you should especially avoid high impact activities like jogging, jumping rope, aerobic dance that requires jumping or springing. Avoid activities that can cause you injuries that would prevent you from doing your daily walking. Accidents that cause long inactivity will cause you to lose much of what you've gained. You need no other exercise activities other than your walking program if you don't want to do any more. It is a good idea to have some other aerobic exercises available to you for those days when you can't walk because of inclement weather or some other preventing problem. Swimming, stationary biking or rowing are ideal. All are good aerobic, low impact activities.

Such activities as tennis, racquet ball, baseball, weight lifting and training or body building, are anaerobic and wonderful activities, if you enjoy them, but remember they do not take the place of your walking program and must be done in addition to your walking. If these activities cause stress and pain to your hips, knees or ankles because of your weight, stay away from them until your joints and muscles become stronger and can compensate for the stresses caused by your weight. Golf and bowling are great social and stress reducing activities and help keep your joints limber, but are neither anaerobic nor aerobic for most of us. Again, if you enjoy them, participate in them in addition to your walking program

6

Detection & Screening

The major purpose of screening for any cancer is to detect the disease at its earliest possible stages, hopefully before any symptoms have developed. However, some men, will experience symptoms that might indicate the presence of prostate cancer, but because these symptoms may also indicate the presence of other diseases or disorders like prostatitis, or BPH, patients may put off examination until the symptoms become too intrusive or uncomfortable. After the age of 40 it is wise to have a prostate evaluation along with your general physical or even once yearly if there are any symptoms at all. Typically, men whose prostate cancer is detected through screening before symptoms arise, are found to have very early-stage disease that can be treated most effectively with higher incidence of cure.

Screening for prostate cancer is performed quickly and easily in a physician's office using two tests: the **PSA** or **Prostate-Specific Antigen**, a blood test, and the **Digital Rectal Exam** or **DRE,** perhaps seen and felt unpleasant to many men, but non-the-less painless.

The PSA Blood Test or PSA

The **PSA** is a protein found in the blood of men, which is produced by the prostate gland and released in very small amounts into the bloodstream. When there's an enlargement of the prostate, as when prostate cancer develops and grows, more PSA is released where it can be detected in the blood. To accomplish the PSA test a small amount of blood is drawn and the level of PSA is measured. PSA levels under 4 ng/mL are usually considered normal, while levels over 10 ng/mL are usually considered excessively high. Results between 4 and 10 ng/mL are usually considered as being questionable or intermediate. A major problem with the PSA is that it can also be elevated if other prostate problems are present, such as BPH or prostatitis, while some men with prostate cancer still may have low levels of PSA. This is why both the PSA and the digital rectal exam or DRE are used together to detect the presence of prostatic cancers.

The Digital Rectal Exam

To perform the digital rectal exam or DRE, the physician inserts a gloved, lubricated finger into the rectum and examines the prostate gland for any irregularities in size, shape, and texture. The prostate is easily felt through the anterior rectal wall abourt half a finger's length past the anal sphincter, making the exam relatively simple and painless but somewhat annoying to most men. The DRE is useful to physicians to help them distinguish between prostate cancer and non-cancerous conditions such as BPH or prostatitis. The American Cancer Society recommends that both the PSA and DRE should be offered annually, beginning at age 50. Men at high risk, such as African American men and men with a strong family history of should begin testing at age 45; however, I feel that all men over 40 should speak with their physicians at the time of their annual physicals and consider including the PSA and/or DRE routinely from 40 on.

What Are Prostate Cancer Symptoms?

Prostate cancer caught at its earliest stages, will rarely produce any symptoms. In these rare cases men may experience symptoms that include:

1. The need to urinate frequently, especially at night.
2. Difficulty starting to urinate or holding back urine.
3. A weak or interrupted flow of urine.
4. Uncomfortable, painful or burning urination.
5. Erectile Dysfunction, ED or difficulty in having an erection;
6. Painful ejaculation.
7. Blood in urine or semen.
8. Frequent pain or stiffness in the lower back, hips, or upper thighs.

The problem raised by these symptoms is that none are cancer specific; all can more often be caused by other benign diseases. Therefore, men who experience any of these symptoms need to undergo a thorough work-up to determine the underlying cause of the symptoms. Fortunately, in most cases the examinations will prove some problem other than cancer, but should cancer be present the earlier the discovery the surer the chances for a cure.

7

The Diagnosis of Prostate Cancer

Neither the Digital Rectal Exam or DRE nor the Prostate Specific Antigen or PSA tests can diagnose prostate cancer, but their value is in that they can signal the need for a ***prostate biopsy*** to examine the prostate cells , which can determine whether they are cancerous. Unexplained changes in urinary or sexual function may lead to a full evaluation by the doctor, and, if prostate cancer is suspected, a biopsy should be performed.? To accomplish a prostate biopsy, needles are inserted into the prostate to take small samples of tissue, usually under the guidance of ultrasound imaging. The biopsy procedure may cause some discomfort or pain, but the procedure is short, and is usually be performed as an office or outpatient procedure.

Gleason Grading and Gleason Scores

Normal prostate gland cells are constantly reproducing and dying, and each new cell has the same appearance as all of the other normal prostate cells. However, cancer cells look different, forming five distinct patterns, and the degree in which they vary from the normal cells determines their cancer grading. This grading is on a continuum between "low-grade" tumor cells, which tend to look very similar to normal cells, and "high-grade" tumor cells that have mutated so drastically that they often barely resemble the normal cells at all.

The Gleason grading system distinguishes these five distinct patterns that prostate tumor cells may go through as they mutate from normal cells. The scale runs from 1 to 5, 1 representing cells that are nearly normal, and 5 representing cells that resemble prostate cells hardly at all.

A pathologist, examining the cells of a prostate biopsy's samples under a microscope, assigns one Gleason grade to the most common pattern, and a second Gleason grade to the next most common pattern. The two grades are added, the sum determining the Gleason score. The Gleason score tends to predict the aggressiveness of the cancer and how it will progress The higher the Gleason score, the more aggressive the tumor tends to be.

Staging the Disease

Staging, on the other hand, determines the extent to which the prostate cancer has progressed. *Localized prostate cancer* means the cancer is confined within the prostate gland itself and has not extended beyond the edge of the gland itself. *Locally advanced prostate cancer* means that most of the cancer is still confined within the prostate, but some has started to escape to or into the immediate surrounding tissues. *In metastatic prostate cancer,* the cancer is growing outside the prostate and its immediate neighboring tissues and possibly spread to more distant organs.

Other test used to determine
stages of prostate cancer

A number of tests may be used to help determine the stage this disease. Often cancers growing outside of the prostate can be detected through traditional imaging studies, such as CT scans, MRIs, or x-rays, and through more specialized imaging like bone scans. However, these tests may not be able to detect very small groups of cancer cells, results of these tests cannot be used alone to determine the stage of the disease. Metastatic disease can also be detected through imaging studies, and may often be detected in the lymph nodes. Cancers cells that spread to distant organs usually travel through the *lymphatic system*, another circulatory system similar to the blood stream carrying cells intended to fight infection and disease. Often during a biopsy, or during surgery, groups of lymph nodes will be removed and examined for the presence of cancer cells. Knowing the stage of disease is important to determine how aggressively the disease should be treated, and how likely it is to be eradicated by the selected treatment options.

8

Treatment

Treatment for prostate cancer I quite variable, each method having its own pros and cons, so each man must in conjunction with his physicians, make his own decision as to which is best for him. The decision will most likely depend on a combination of clinical and psychological factors. Consideration of these different options is the first step to deciding on the best treatment course. Start with a consultation with the three types of prostate cancer specialists, a urologist, a radiation oncologist and a medical oncologist. They will, in combination, offer the most comprehensive evaluation of the available treatments and their expected outcomes.

Active Surveillance

The concept of active surveillance, or prudent and watchful waiting, has become a frequently selected option for men who have decided not to undergo immediate surgery, chemo or radiation therapy. During this active surveillance period, the cancer is carefully monitored for signs of progression. A PSA blood test and DRE or Digital Rectal Exam are usually administered every six months with a recommended yearly biopsy of the prostate. If symptoms develop, or if tests indicate that the cancer is growing, treatment must be reconsidered. Active surveillance might be a good choice for men who have very slow growing, very early cancers, or men who have other serious medical conditions, which might be affected by cancer treatments.

Prostatectomy

Removal of the prostate gland is a surgical approach toward the treatment of prostate cancer. This may involve removal of all or part of the prostate gland. Men with early-stage cancer that is confined to the prostate and not any surrounding tissues, will undergo radical prostatectomy. Radical prostatectomy is surgical removal of the entire prostate gland plus some surrounding tissue. At the most common type of prostatectomy, a *radical retropubic prostatectomy*, an incision is made in the lower abdomen and the prostate is taken out from behind the pubic bone. After the prostate is successfully removed, the surgeon stitches the urethra directly to the bladder so urine is able to flow normally out of the bladder and body.

In a nerve-sparing prostatectomy, the surgeon makes every attempt to cuts to the very edges of the prostate, taking care to spare the erectile nerves that run alongside the prostate. In those situations where these nerves cannot be spared due to the extent of the cancer going beyond the prostate, surgically grafting nerves from other parts of the body to the ends of the cut erectile nerves might be possible.

Laparoscopic surgery has made it possible in some cases to do the surgery through very small incisions made in the abdomen, through which the surgeon inserts narrow instruments fitted with cameras and surgical tools, allowing the visualization and removal of the cancerous structures without cutting open the entire abdomen.

Surgical Procedures for Advanced and Recurrent Prostate Cancers

About 30% of men predicted *"cured"* with their initial treatment for early-stage prostate cancer will relapse after five years. For these men, and for those diagnosed with advanced-stage disease, surgical techniques other than radical prostatectomy may be advised for treatment of their prostate cancer management. Those men who underwent **radiation therapy** as initial therapy might benefit from a *"salvage prostatectomy"* In this procedure, the prostate and its surrounding tissues, including the tissues previously irradiated, are removed. However, even under the best of circumstances, post-radiation surgery may be a very difficult operation and might result in significant side effects.

The best outcomes For surgical and radiation are seen in those men whose PSA levels are low and whose disease has not spread too far. Regular monitoring of PSA levels after primary therapy must be performed and is key successful treatment, as is prompt initiation of treatment upon disease recurrence.

Radiation Therapy

Radiation Therapy for Advanced or Recurrent Prostate Cancer

Men who previously underwent prostatectomy, external beam radiation can be delivered to the area immediately surrounding where the prostate was, this in the hopes of eradicating any remaining prostate cells that may have been left behind. It must be noted that effects of the radiation therapy can be moderately severe, and would be additive to those previously received with surgery. As for men who previously have undergone external beam radiation therapy, **brachytherapy,** or radioactive seed implantation, can provide additional tumor control. Again, the best outcomes are seen in those men whose PSA levels are low and whose disease has not spread too far. Regular monitoring of PSA levels after primary therapy and prompt initiation of treatment upon disease recurrence is key to survival; the earlier the treatment is begun, the better the likelihood of improved results. External beam radiation therapy is also a possible option in men with painful bone metastases.

Bone metastasis from prostate cancer

When prostate cancer cells spread to the bones they are known as **prostate cancer bone metastases** rather than bone cancer. Once in the bones, the prostate cancer cells multiply and start to impede the normal health and strength of the affected bones, leading to bone pain, fracture, or other complications and health problems. Early detection of bone metastases influences the type and success of treatment. Men with prostate cancer bone metastases frequently experience painful episodes; pain management is an important part of all treatment strategies.

Chemotherapy

Chemotherapy refers to therapy that uses chemicals to kill, halt, or slow the growth of cancer cells. Chemotherapy drugs work in various ways, but are all based on stopping the cancer cells from dividing thus stopping the growth and further spread or invasion of the tumor.

Chemotherapy can take a toll on the body. The fact is that the FDA has approved few chemotherapy drugs for use in treating prostate cancer. However, over the years, doctors have found some chemo drugs designed for used in other types of cancers that can be used effectively with prostate cancer. The use of a drug designed to treat one disease for the treatment of another affliction is known as *off label use of a drug.* Off label use of chemotherapy drugs is common in the treatment of men with prostate cancer.

Other Treatment Options

Radiation therapy and surgery remain the gold standard for treatment of localized prostate cancer, but other, less popular treatment options might be beneficial as well. The below listed are a few being used.

Cryotherapy

In cryotherapy, also known as cryosurgery or cryoablation, probes are inserted into the prostate glad and argon gas or liquid nitrogen is delivered to the prostate, literally freezing to death the prostate cells and any prostate tumors. Care must be taken to avoid freezing damage to the nearby structures. With this type treatment the incidence for both erectile and urinary dysfunction remain high. Data on long-term outcomes are limited for cryotherapy. Cryotherapy may also be used as a secondary local therapy in men who have undergone radiation therapy as their initial treatment for early-stage prostate cancer.

High-Intensity Focused Ultrasound

With *High-Intensity Focused Ultrasound*, also known as *HIFU*, the prostate cells are heated until they are heat killed. An ultrasound probe is inserted into the rectum and then aims very high-intensity ultrasound waves, which are delivered to the target area. This technique has been used in Europe for several years with considerable success, however it still remains experimental in the United States.

Primary Hormone Therapy

Hormone therapy, known as *androgen-deprivation therapy* or *ADT*, is intended to stop testosterone from being released and prevent the hormone from acting on the prostate cells. Though there is little, data showing that hormone therapy alone is an effective treatment strategy for men with localized prostate cancer, it is being increasingly used in such cases as a middle ground between active surveillance and local therapy.

Continuing research

A tremendous amount of research in the detection and treatment of prostate cancer is ongoing worldwide and is showing optimistic results. However, whatever the future for treatment will be, the fact that *most* prostate cancer has its onset in a man's later years of life and is also *usually* slow growing, any one diagnosed with the disease today will probably not die of his prostate cancer. There is a usually true saying, "Most men with prostate cancer will die *with* their disease but *not from* their disease!"

9

Managing Bone Metastases and Pain

As mentioned before, prostate cancer cells that spread to the bone are known as *prostate cancer bone metastases* rather than bone cancer. These prostate cancer cells, once settled into bones, begin to interfere with the normal health and strength of the bones, often leading to bone pain, fractures, or other complications. Early detection of bone metastases can help to determine the best treatment strategy, and often ward off complications caused by the metastases.

Detecting Prostate Cancer Metastases

When they spread prostate cancer cells tend to settle first locally, in the nearby pelvic bone, the lower spine, and the upper thighs. Often men first experience pelvic area pain as a sign that the cancer might have spread to bone. Detection tools can be used to pinpoint the location of the metastases in order to better assess how to treat them. The bone scan is the "gold standard" test for locating bone metastases. This test procedure utilizes a radioactive substance, which acts like a dye injected in a vein. Then images of the entire skeleton are taken and the radioactive dye-like material, shows where bone tissue is rapidly changing, a characteristic effect of prostate cancer bone metastases.

Though bone scans can detect even very small amounts of increased bone metabolism, it must be noted that not all such changes are caused by prostate cancer bone metastases. The radioactive dye might be detecting changes a bone due to a previous fracture, infection, arthritis, or even bone loss that can result from the use of hormone therapy. In addition other types of tests, such as x-rays, CT scans, MRIs, and PET scans, are typically used to further monitor the effects of the metastases over time.

Treating Metastases
Radiation Therapy Targeting
Bone Metastases?

Radiation targeted directly to the metastasis will often be a major treatment method. This will kill the prostate cancer cells, slow or end growth and relieve the pain. This external beam radiation therapy, sometimes referred to as spot radiation uses targeted x-rays to kill the cancer cells that have settled in the bones. Radiation oncologists map out very precisely the cancer cell area to ensure that the x-rays are targeting the metastasis and are not causing damage to the surrounding bone and muscle tissue.

Radiopharmacology

Radiopharmaceuticals are radioactive drugs that are injected into the body through a vein and settle in the bone metastases. There they release radiation to the local area and kill the cancer cells. This treatment is often used in combination with other chemotherapy.

Bone-Targeting Agents known as Bisphosphonates

Bone cells are normally destroyed and created at a constant rate. Osteoblasts are cells that form new bone cells. Their activity if unchecked would ultimately results in an overgrowth of bone tissue. Osteoclasts are cells that destroy bone cells and if unchecked would ultimately results in porous, brittle bone tissue. In men with prostate cancer bone metastases, both of these processes occur at accelerated rates, leading to both an overgrowth of bone tissue and weakened and brittle bones. The combination of these two processes makes the bones unstable and prone to fracture. *Bisphosphonates* are drugs designed to help reestablish and maintain the proper balance in the *normal* bone growth and bone destruction. The bisphosphonate *Zoledronic acid (Zometa)* is often given intravenously at the onset of prostate cancer bone metastases and can delay the onset of complications and relieve pain. It is given once every three weeks in a 15-minute infusion.

Oral bisphosphonates are also available and may be used in men with prostate cancer to prevent or slow bone loss while taking hormone therapy. These drugs, *alendronate (Fosamax)* and *risedronate (Actonel),* are given in pill form.

Other than fractures of the weakened bones, the most significant complication from bone metastases is spinal cord compression. Weakening of vertebra by prostate cancer bone metastasis may result in the weakened bones of the spinal column collapsing and compressing the spinal cord housed within the bones or the nerves that run out between them. Such cord or nerve compression can cause severe nerve damage, pain, weaknesses, and possibly paralysis.

Managing Pain

Pain management is an extremely important part of prostate cancer and prostate cancer bone metastases treatment. Physicians may select any umber of pain medications and should not withhold such treatment. Some patients may require mild and over the counter medications while others may require prescription drugs and narcotics. A physician, keeping in mind that every pain medication has its own set of side effects, should closely monitor pain treatments. The most common side effect of pain medication use is constipation. Other side effects may include dizziness, impaired balance, falling, nausea and vomiting, sleepiness, and confusion. These side effects have to be addressed on a case-by-case situation.

In addition

It is an important during treatment of prostate cancer bone metastases management to maintain adequate calcium and vitamin D levels. Also exercising regularly is of extreme benefit. Both will help to maintain bone strength and help to minimize bone loss and osteoporosis, which can make treating bone metastases more challenging.

10

What to Consider When Your PSA Rises After Initial Treatment

After a surgical prostatectomy the most widely accepted suggestion of a recurrence of prostate cancer is a PSA that has risen on at least two separate occasions at least two weeks apart, measured by the same lab. In the post-radiation therapy setting, the most widely accepted definition is a PSA that has risen from it's all-time low in at least three consecutive tests conducted at least two weeks apart, measured by the same lab. It's important to always use the same lab for all of your tests as PSA values may fluctuate significantly from lab to lab. The rate at which your PSA rises, can be a significant factor in determining is the aggressiveness of your recurrent cancer.

Regular monitoring of PSA levels after primary therapy is key, as is prompt initiation of treatment upon disease recurrence. The earlier the treatment is begun, the better the likelihood of improved results.

If your PSA starts to rise after you've undergone prostatectomy, *salvage radiation therapy* might be considered as a follow-up therapy. In this treatment external beam radiation is delivered to the area immediately surrounding where the prostate was, to eradicate any remaining prostate cells having been left behind.

After initial radiation therapy surgical follow-up or *"salvage" prostatectomy* may be considered. Surgeons at some of the larger cancer centers have been seeing improved results with post radiation surgery, but even under the best of circumstances, post-radiation surgery is a very difficult operation to perform, and few surgeons across the country perform it regularly.

Androgen deprivation therapy or *"hormone therapy"* is frequently a key treatment strategy for recurrent prostate cancer following other local treatment. The goal hormone therapies is to stop the production and interfere with the effects of testosterone which fuels the growth of the prostate cancer cells. However, not all prostate cancer cells are sensitive to increases or decreases in testosterone levels, therefore hormone therapy is an ancillary treatment for prostate cancer but does not cure the disease. Approaches to blocking the secretion of testosterone include the surgical removal of the testes, drugs known as *LHRH agonists*, and the administration of estrogens. *Antiandrogens* may be used to block the action of testosterone by preventing its active form known as *DHT* from entering the central part of the prostate cancer cell; without DHT, the growth of prostate cancer cells is prevented.

Patients should review the side effects of the different hormone therapy regimens with their physicians, and discuss ways to minimize their side effects. It's very important that you understand the value of the therapy selected to manage your prostate cancer, but also that you learn how to live your life the best way possible while fighting the disease.

Glossary

ablation: The removal or destruction of a body part or tissue or its function. Surgery, hormones, drugs, radio frequency, heat, or other methods may perform ablation.

adjuvant: Any additional treatment used to increase the effectiveness of the primary therapy.

adjuvant therapy: Treatment given after the primary treatment to increase the chances of a cure. Adjuvant therapy may include chemotherapy, radiation therapy, hormone therapy, post radiation or post chemo surgery, or biological therapy.

adrenal gland: Two small glands, one located on top of each kidney, that produce steroid hormones, adrenaline, and nor-adrenaline, which help control heart rate, blood pressure, and other important body functions. There are two adrenal glands,

analog: In chemistry, this is a substance that is similar, but not identical, to another.

androgen: A hormone that promotes the development and maintenance of male sex characteristics.

anti-androgen: A drug used to block the production or interfere with the action of male sex hormones or androgens.

anti-androgen withdrawal response: A decrease in PSA caused by the withdrawal of an anti-androgen such as Casodex or flutamide after CHT begins to fail.

—B—

benign: Not cancerous; benign tumors do not spread to tissues around them or to other parts of the body.

benign prostatic hyperplasia or hypertrophy (BPH): BPH is a benign (non-cancerous) condition in which an overgrowth of prostate tissue may push against the urethra and the bladder, blocking the flow of urine.

bilateral: Affecting both the right and left sides of the body.

biopsy: The removal of cells or tissues for examination under a microscope. An incisional biopsy or core biopsy is one in which only a sample of tissue is removed, while an excisional biopsy is when an entire lump or suspicious area is removed. When a sample of tissue or fluid is withdrawn through a needle, the procedure is called a needle biopsy or fine-needle aspiration.

bone scan: A technique to create images of bones on a computer screen or on film by infusing a small amount of radioactive material into a blood vessel, which then travels through the bloodstream to be collects in the bones and detected by a scanner.

brachytherapy: A procedure in which a radioactive material sealed in needles, seeds, wires, or catheters is placed directly into or near a tumor; it may also be called internal radiation, implant radiation, or interstitial radiation therapy.

—D—

deoxyribonucleic acid (DNA): The molecules inside cells that carry genetic information and pass it from one generation to the next.

DHT: See dihydrotestosterone

differentiation: In cancer, refers to how maturely developed cancer cells are in a tumor. Differentiated tumor cells resemble normal cells and tend to grow and spread at a slower rate than undifferentiated or poorly differentiated tumor cells.

digital rectal examination (DRE): An examination in which a doctor inserts a lubricated, gloved finger into the rectum to feel for prostatic abnormalities.

dihydrotestosterone (DHT): Also known as 5-alpha-dihydrotestosterone, is the male hormone which is active in the prostate; it is made when an enzyme 5-alpha-reductase transforms testosterone to DHT which stimulates the growth of prostate tissue.

double-blind, double-blinded: A clinical trial in which neither the medical staff nor the test person knows which of several possible therapies the person is receiving.

downsizing, downstaging: The use of hormonal, radiation, chemo, or other forms of management to reduce the volume of prostate cancer in and/or around the prostate prior to other attempted curative treatment.

duct: A tube or vessel of the body through which fluids pass.

dysplasia: Cells that look abnormal under a microscope but are not cancer; dysplasia may be precancerous.

—E—

EBR, EBRT: External Beam Radiation Therapy.

ejaculation: The ejection of semen through the penis during orgasm.

endorectal: Approached through the rectum, such as endorectal MRIs or transrectal ultrasound (TRUS), ultrasound to visualize the area.

endorectal ultrasound (ERUS): A procedure in which a probe that sends out high-energy sound waves is inserted into the rectum. The echoes form a picture of body tissue called a sonogram.

epithelium: Skin and other thin layer of tissue that cover organs, glands, and structures within the body.

erectile dysfunction (ED): An inability to have an erection adequate for sexual intercourse.

estrogen: A hormone that promotes the development and maintenance of female sexual characteristics.

EXBT, EXRT: External beam therapy; external radiation therapy in which the radiation is delivered by a machine pointed at the area to be radiated; it may also be known as external beam radiation (EBR, XBR), external beam radiation therapy (EBRT, XBRT).

—F—

Finasteride: A drug used to reduce the amount of male hormone testosterone produced by the body, often used to shrink the hypertrophic prostate gland.

fine-needle aspiration: The removal of tissue or fluid with a needle for examination in the lab under a microscope, and may also be called needle biopsy.

flare: A sudden initial reaction when starting hormone therapy, may be characterized by severe increase in symptoms, such as pain; does not occur in all men and may be prevented by taking an anti-androgen like Casodex, Nilandron prior to starting hormone therapy.

Flutamide: An anticancer drug belonging to the family of drugs called anti-androgens.

free PSA or fPSA: PSA exists in two forms, either bound to protein or unbound, the "free" form; by measuring both the bound and free form can better predict risk.

—G—

gastrointestinal (GI): Refers to the stomach and intestines, the digestive and excretory system.

gland: An organ that makes one or more substances such as hormones, digestive juices, sweat, tears, saliva, or milk. Glands are of two types; endocrine glands, which release their secretion substances directly into the bloodstream, and exocrine glands that release the secretions into a duct or opening to the inside or outside of the body.

Gleason Score (GS)- Gleason Grade: A system of grading prostate cancer cells based on how they look under a microscope. Gleason scores range from 2 to 10 to help indicate how likely it will be that a tumor will spread, a low Gleason score meaning the cancer cells are similar to normal prostate cells and are less likely to spread; a high Gleason score means the cancer cells are very different from normal and are more likely to spread.

gonads: The part of the reproductive system that produces and releases eggs in women, the ovaries, or sperm in men, the testis.

gonadotropin-releasing hormone (GnRH): A hormone made by the hypothalamus in the brain. GnRH causes the pituitary gland to make luteinizing hormone (LH) and follicle stimulating hormone (FSH), hormones involved in reproduction.

Goserelin: A drug that belongs to the family of drugs called gonadotropin-releasing hormone analogs, used to block hormone production in the ovaries or testicles.

goserelin acetate: Zoladex, a luteinizing hormone-releasing hormone (LHRH) analog used in the palliative hormonal treatment of advanced prostate cancer and in the adjuvant hormonal treatment of earlier stages of prostate cancer..

grade: The grade of a tumor depends on how abnormal the cancer cells look under a microscope and may be used to estimate how quickly the tumor is likely to grow and spread.

grading: A system for classifying cancer cells in terms of how abnormal they appear under a microscope; the objective being to provide a predictor about the probable growth rate of the tumor and its tendency to spread and plays a role in treatment decisions.

—**H**—

high-dose-rate (HDR): An internal radiation treatment in which the radioactive source is removed between treatments.

high-dose-rate remote brachytherapy: An internal radiation treatment in which the radioactive source is removed between treatments. Also called high-dose-rate remote radiation therapy or remote brachytherapy.

histology: The study of tissues and cells under a microscope.

hormone: A chemical made by glands within the body that circulate in the bloodstream and controlling the actions of certain cells or organs.

hormone antagonists: Chemical substances which inhibit the function of the endocrine glands, the production of their secreted hormones, or the action of hormones upon their specific sites.

hormone refractory prostate cancer: Prostate cancer that has become refractory, and resists hormone therapy.

hormone therapy (HT): Treatment that adds, blocks, or removes hormones to slow or stop the growth of certain cancers, such as prostate and breast cancer, synthetic hormones or other drugs may be given to block the body's natural hormones.

HRPC: Hormone refractory prostate cancer are prostate cancers that resists hormone therapy.

hyperplasia: An abnormal increase in the number of cells in an organ or tissue.

hypertrophy: The enlargement or overgrowth of an organ due to an increase in size of its constituent cells.

—I—

IAS: Intermittent androgen suppression; the starting and stopping of the treatment.

ICHT: Intermittent combined hormone therapy; the starting and stopping of treatment.

IHT: Intermittent hormone therapy; the starting and stopping of treatment.

immunoassay: A test that uses the binding of antibodies to antigens to identify and measure certain substances.

impotency: In medicine, refers to the inability to have an erection of the penis adequate for sexual intercourse or erectile dysfunction.

incontinence: The inability to control the flow of urine from the bladder (urinary incontinence) or the escape of stool from the rectum (fecal incontinence).

insulin: A hormone made by the islet cells of the pancreas and controls the amount of sugar in the blood by moving it into the cells, where it can be used by the body for energy.

intensity modulated radiation therapy (IMRT): A type of 3-dimensional radiation therapy that uses computer-generated images to show the size and shape of the tumor, so thin beams of radiation of different intensities can be aimed at a tumor from many angles, so as to reduces the damage to healthy tissue near the tumor.

interstitial: Situated between parts or in the interspaces of a tissue.

interstitial radiation therapy (IRT): A procedure in which radioactive material sealed in needles, seeds, wires, or catheters is placed directly into or near a tumor, and may also be called brachytherapy, internal radiation, or implant radiation.

intraepithelial: Within the layer of cells that form the surface or lining of an organ.

—J—

Jewett staging system: A staging system for prostate cancer that uses ABCD; "A" and "B" refer to cancer that is confined to the prostate, "C" refers to cancer that has grown out of the prostate but has not spread to lymph nodes or other places in the body. "D" refers to cancer that has spread to lymph nodes or to other places in the body. This system is also called the ABCD rating or the Whitmore-Jewett staging system.

—L—

laparoscopy: The insertion of a thin, lighted tube, called a laparoscope, through a small incision, in a joint or the abdominal wall to inspect the inside of a joint or the abdomen and remove tissue samples.

leuprolide: A drug that belongs to a family of drugs called gonadotropin-releasing hormone analogs, used to block hormone production in the ovaries or testicles.

libido: The level of interest in sexual activity.

luteinizing hormone (LH): The pituitary hormone that causes the testicles in men and ovaries in women to manufacture hormones.

luteinizing hormone-releasing hormone (LHRH): A hormone that stimulates the production of sex hormones in men and women.

lymph: The clear fluid that travels through the lymphatic system and carries cells that help fight infections and other diseases.

lymph nodes: A rounded mass of lymphatic tissue that filter lymphatic fluid, and store lymphocytes white blood cells and are located along lymphatic vessels. Also called a lymph gland.

lymphatic system: The tissues and organs that produce, store, and carry white blood cells that fight infections and other diseases; this system includes the bone marrow, spleen, thymus, lymph nodes, and lymphatic vessels, a network of thin tubes that carry lymph and white blood cells, like blood vessels, into all the tissues of the body.

lymphocyte: A type of white blood cell that have a number of roles in the immune system, including the production of antibodies and other substances that fight infection and diseases.

—M—

magnetic resonance imaging (MRI): A procedure in which radio waves and a powerful magnet linked to a computer are used to create detailed pictures of areas inside the body, and can show the difference between normal and diseased tissue. The MRI makes better images of organs and soft tissue than other scanning techniques, such as CT or X-ray. MRI is especially useful for imaging the brain, spine, the soft tissue of joints, and the inside of bones.

malignant: Cancerous, malignant tumors can invade and destroy nearby tissue and spread to other parts of the body.

marker: A diagnostic indication that disease may develop.

metastasis: The spread of cancer from one part of the body to another; a tumor formed by cells that have spread is called a "metastatic tumor" or a "metastasis." The metastatic tumor contains cells that are like those in the original (primary) tumor.

morbidity: A disease or the incidence of disease within a population; morbidity may also refers to adverse effects caused by a treatment.

—N—

neoadjuvant therapy: Treatment given before the primary treatment. Examples of neoadjuvant therapy include chemotherapy, radiation therapy, and hormone therapy.

neoplasia: Abnormal and uncontrolled cell growth.

nerve sparing: The surgical technique during a prostatectomy where one or both of the neurovascular bundles controlling erections are spared; governed by the extent of the cancer and the skill of the surgeon.

non-steroidal anti-inflammatory drug (NSAID): A drug that decreases fever, inflammation, swelling, pain, and redness.

—O—

oncologist: A physician specializing in treating cancer. Some oncologists specialize in a particular type of cancer treatment, such as, a radiation oncologist specializes in treating cancer with radiation.

orchiectomy: Surgical removal of one or both testicles.

osteoporosis: A condition that is characterized by a decrease in bone mass and density, causing bones to become fragile.

—P—

palliative: Treatment designed to produce relief from symptoms without curing the disease.

palliative care: Care given to improve the quality of life of patients who have a serious or life-threatening disease. The goal of palliative care is to prevent or treat the symptoms of the disease, side effects caused by treatment of the disease, and psychological, social, and spiritual problems related to the disease or its treatment.

palpable: Capable of being felt during a physical examination.

palpable disease: A term used to describe cancer that can be felt by touch, usually present in lymph nodes, skin, or other organs of the body.

Partin Tables: These are tables constructed on the basis of the PSA, stage, grade, and surgical findings of over 4,000 men, and are used to predict the probability that the prostate cancer has spread to the lymph nodes and/or seminal vesicles, penetrated the capsule, or remains confined to the prostate.

pathologist: A physician who identifies diseases by studying cells and tissues under a microscope.

patient-controlled analgesia (PCA): A method in which the patient controls the amount of pain medicine that is used by pressing a button on a computerized pump that is connected to a small tube in the body.

PCa: Abbreviation for prostate cancer.

penis: The external male reproductive organ, which contains a tube called the urethra, which carries semen and urine to the outside of the body.

phase I trial: The first step in testing a new treatment in humans. These studies test for the best ways to give a new treatment, by mouth, intravenous infusion, or injection as well as the best dosing. The dose is usually increased a little at a time in order to find the highest dose that does not cause harmful side effects

phase II trial: Studies to test whether a new treatment has an anticancer effect; for example, whether it shrinks a tumor, improves blood test results, and whether it works against a certain type of cancer.

phase III trial: Studies to compare the results of people taking a new treatment with the results of people taking the standard treatment; which group has better survival rates or fewer side effects. In most cases, studies move into phase III only after a treatment seems to work in phases II and I.

phase IV trial: After a treatment has been approved and is being marketed, it is studied in a phase IV trial to evaluate side effects that were not apparent in the phase III trial.

placebo: An inactive substance or treatment that looks the same as an active drug or treatment being tested; the effects of the active drug or treatment are then compared to the effects of the placebo.

positron emission tomography scan (PET Scan):
A procedure in which a small amount of radioactive glucose is injected into a vein, and a scanner is used to make detailed, computerized pictures of areas inside the body where the glucose is used. Cancer cells tend to use more glucose than normal cells, the scan can be used to find cancer cells in the body.

progesterone: A female hormone.

prognosis: The likely outcome or course of a disease or cancer; the chance of recovery or recurrence.

progression: Increase in the growth size of a tumor or spread of cancer in the body.

Proscar: The brand name of a drug using finasteride that reportedly shrinks the prostate gland in the treatment of BPH and PCa.

Prostascint scan: A scan involving the injection of a radio-labeled antibody that attaches itself to lesions or tumors and can then be visualized on the scan.

prostate gland: A gland in the male reproductive system just below the bladder and surrounds part of the urethra, the canal that empties the bladder, and produces a fluid that forms part of semen.

prostatectomy: An operation to remove part or all of the prostate gland.

prostate-specific antigen (PSA): A substance produced by the prostate that may be found in an increased amount in the blood of men who have prostate cancer, benign prostatic hyperplasia, or infection or inflammation of the prostate gland.

prostatic: Pertaining to the prostate gland.

prostatic acid phosphatase (PAP): An enzyme produced by the prostate, which may be found in increased amounts in men who have prostate cancer.

—R—

radical prostatectomy: Surgery to remove the entire prostate. Gland; two types of radical prostatectomy are retropubic prostatectomy and perineal prostatectomy.

radiography: Producing an image by radiation.

radiolabeled: A compound that has been joined with a radioactive substance.

radiotherapy: The use of high-energy radiation from X-rays, gamma rays, neutrons, and other sources to kill cancer cells and shrink tumors. Radiation may come from a machine outside the body, known as external beam radiation therapy, or from radioactive material placed in the body near cancer cells called internal radiation therapy, implant radiation, or brachytherapy.

rectum: The last several inches of the large intestine ending at the anus.

red blood cell (RBC): A cell that carries oxygen to all parts of the body.

refractory: A disease or condition that does not respond to treatment.

regression: A decrease in the size of a tumor or the extent of cancer in the body.

relapse: The return of signs and symptoms of cancer after a period of improvement.

remission: A decrease in or disappearance of signs and symptoms of cancer.

resection: Surgical removal of part or all of an organ.

resectoscope: An instrument inserted through the urethra and used by a urologist to cut out tissue, usually from the prostate, allowing the physician to actually see precisely where he is cutting.

retention of urine: The inability to completely empty the bladder.

—S—

screening: Checking for diseases when there are no symptoms.

seed, seeding: The implantation of radioactive seeds or pellets, which emit low energy radiation in order to kill surrounding tissue, e.g., the prostate, including prostate cancer cells. Also known as "seed implantation" or "SI" and Brachytherapy,

SEER: Part of the National Cancer Institute for the Surveillance, Epidemiology, and Ends Results Program that maintains statistics on cancer in the US.

semen: The fluid that is released through the penis during orgasm and is made up of sperm from the testicles and fluid from the prostate and other sex glands.

seminal vesicle: A small gland that helps produce semen.

side effect: A problem that occurs when treatment affects tissues or organs other than the target ones being treated, such as fatigue, pain, nausea, vomiting, decreased blood cell counts, hair loss, and mouth sores.

stage, staging: Labeling the extent of a cancer within the body; if the cancer has spread, the stage describes how far it has spread from the original site to other parts of the body.

steroid: A type of drug often used to relieve swelling and inflammation.

—T—

testicle: One of two egg-shaped glands found inside the scrotum that produce sperm and male hormones, also called a testis.

testis, testes: Medical term for testicle. One of two male reproductive glands located inside the scrotum behind and below the penis, which produce sperm and are the primary source of the male hormone testosterone, the plural being "testes."

testosterone: A hormone that promotes the development and maintenance of the male sex characteristics.

TNM staging system: A system for describing the extent of cancer in a patient's body; T describes the size of the tumor and whether it has invaded nearby tissue, N describes any lymph nodes that are involved, and M describes metastasis spread of cancer from one body part to another.

tomography: A series of detailed pictures of areas inside the body created by a computer linked to an x-ray machine.

transrectal ultrasound (TRUS): A procedure in which a probe sending out high-energy sound waves is inserted into the rectum. The sound waves are bounced off internal tissues or organs and make echoes that form a picture of body tissue called a sonogram. TRUS is used to look for abnormalities in the rectum and nearby structures, including the prostate.

transurethral prostatectomy: Also called a transurethral resection of the prostate or TURP performed with a special instrument inserted through the urethra.

transurethral resection of the prostate (TURP): Surgical procedure to remove excessive tissue from the prostate using an instrument inserted through the urethra.

tumor: A mass of excess tissue that results from abnormal cell division that perform no useful body function and may be benign (not cancerous) or malignant (cancerous).

—U—

ultrasound (US): A procedure in which high-energy sound waves (ultrasound) are bounced off internal tissues or organs and make echoes, which form a picture of body tissues called a sonogram. Also called ultrasonography.

ureter: The tube that carries urine from the kidney to the bladder.

urethra: The tube through which urine leaves the body from the bladder.

—W—

watchful waiting (WW): Closely monitoring a patient's condition but withholding treatment until symptoms appear or change. Also called observation.

Whitmore-Jewett staging system: A staging system for prostate cancer that uses ABCD; "A" and "B" refer to cancer that is confined to the prostate, "C" refers to cancer that has grown out of the prostate but has not spread to lymph nodes or other places in the body, and "D" refers to cancer that has spread to lymph nodes or to other places in the body. Also called the ABCD rating or the Jewett staging system.

—Z—

Zoladex: Trade or brand name for goserelin acetate, an LHRH used in hormone therapy.

In dealing with Prostate Cancer, as with any other cancer, achieving and maintaining good health is a prime importance. Smoking is by far one of the most devastating habits to good health. If you smoke STOP! If you live with a smoker or work among smokers you must stay away form their side stream smoke. The following program is provided for you or your loved ones to end this deadly habit.

QUIT SMOKING NOW™ is a program to help you break your smoking addiction. As with any other addiction, it is important you admit you have an addiction to tobacco products. Denial is the biggest obstacle to breaking your addiction to tobacco use.

Quit Smoking Now! ™

The Program to Help You Quit Smoking Now and Forever!

by
Othniel J. Seiden, MD
&
Jane L. Bilett, PhD

The free (or nearly free) version of this book is sponsored by Doctors to the World in support of the
CLEAN INDOOR AIR COALITION (CIAC).

Dedicated to
All the non-smokers of the world
who've every right to breathe clean air

and to those ready to kick
their addiction to tobacco products.

WHY COLD TURKEY?

Because tobacco use is an addiction, the best way to "kick" your habit is to quit "cold turkey." That may sound difficult and cruel and may intimidate you, but kicking cold turkey is indeed the best way to quit smoking. In fact, over 90% of all those who successfully become non-smokers did it cold turkey.

Why is cold turkey the best way to stop smoking? Smoking is an addiction to the chemical, Nicotine. As with any addiction, tapering off only keeps the addiction alive. No one who has had experience in alcohol addiction treatment would ever suggest tapering off booze. Each drink only increases the desire or need to continue drinking. The same is true of smoking. Each smoke makes your body crave another smoke. Tapering off only prolongs the agony and strengthens the addiction.

THE "KICK COLD TURKEY" CEREMONY!

It is important that you make a hard commitment to quit your smoking habit. You have to make an investment in quitting. One way to do this is to get rid of all your smoking paraphernalia. After all, if you are committed to quitting, you certainly don't need to keep anything related to smoking. If you're not willing to get rid of your smoking paraphernalia, you obviously aren't too serious about becoming a non-smoker for the rest of your life. That is, after all what it means to quit smoking ... becoming a non-smoker for the rest of your life.

Non-smokers do not need smoking paraphernalia.

Non-smokers do not need ashtrays, humidors, pipes, pipe cleaners, tobacco, cigars, cigarette, lighters, tobacco pouches, snuff, chewing tobacco, cuspidors, etc., etc., etc.

The "Kick Cold Turkey" ceremony is where you get rid of all these trappings. It means that if you ever go back to smoking you'll have to make an active decision to reinvest in smoking supplies and that may, in itself, be just enough of a deterrent to keep you from "falling off the wagon!"

Gather everything that is part of your smoking habit and throw it into the trash.

If you hold back, you are only hurting yourself. **THE MORE YOU GET RID OF, THE GREATER YOUR COMMITMENT, AND THE BETTER YOUR CHANCES FOR SUCCESS.**

When Othniel Seiden (the author of this text) quit, he gave away a brand new box of cigars with only one of them smoked. That was about a $50.00 commitment. In addition, he got rid of a humidor and about seven pipes, an additional $180.00 commitment. He also cleaned his home and office of all ashtrays, lighters and smoking gadgetry which brought his total commitment up to roughly $280.00. By the time, his wife had all the drapes and furniture cleaned of the smoke residue and smell, his investment in quitting topped $550.00. Believe him when he tells you... that made it difficult to consider a return to smoking.

Your success in quitting makes the sacrifice of all that paraphernalia well worthwhile. On the other hand, to revert to smoking, you would suddenly realize you wasted the entire investment of discards.

Now that you have discarded your smoking paraphernalia, you are a non-smoker!

Congratulations!
YOU ARE A NON-SMOKER!

IT IS IMPORTANT THAT YOU THINK OF YOURSELF AS A NON-SMOKER! REALIZE IT ... YOU ARE A NON-SMOKER!

SMOKING OR ANY OTHER TOBACCO USE IS AN ADDICTION!

Let's reemphasize, "Smoking or tobacco use is an addiction!" Smoking is an addiction to the chemical substance *Nicotine*. Nicotine addiction is considered by many authorities to be as strong as an addiction to heroin or opium. That being the case, now is the best time to quit because **tomorrow your addiction will be stronger.**

Don't let the addiction facts intimidate you.

The half-life of nicotine in your system is relatively short and addiction withdrawal to nicotine is usually over within 48 hours. In fact, it is not the physical withdrawal that will likely cause you the greatest difficulty in quitting. There are two other factors involved with smoking in addition to addiction which you must understand; they are psychological dependence and habituation. Let's take a more detailed look at the differences between addiction, psychological dependence and habituation.

ADDICTION...

Addiction involves an actual biologic physical craving by the cells of your body for the chemical substance nicotine. Nicotine is found only in tobacco in an additive state. The longer and more frequently you use tobacco products in any form, the stronger your addiction becomes. The stronger your addiction becomes, the more intense your withdrawal symptoms are likely to be. Once you are addicted to nicotine, you are always addicted to nicotine. That does not mean that you never get over the withdrawal symptoms; you'll get over those in a relatively short time and may suffer surprisingly few ill effects.

What it means to be, **"Once an addict, always an addict,"** is that if you ever indulge yourself in a tobacco product you'll be immediately "hooked" again and at the same level as you were when you quit. It is very important that you realize this. If you smoked two packs a day, and you quit for twenty or more years, and you try a smoke twenty or more years from now, within a day or two of that first smoke *you will probably be back to two or more packs a day!* Your addiction is no different from that of an alcoholic or a hard drug junkie. One drink and an alcoholic will go right back to being a drunk ... one snort and a coke head will go right back to being a hard drug user ... and one smoke, chew or snuff and you'll be right back to the habit level you just left. That is what addiction means. You are a tobacco addict and you must never forget it! This is not a moral judgment but statement of a physical and biological fact. Addiction will not be a problem for you unless you expose yourself to the ingestion of nicotine at some time in the future.

PSYCHOLOGICAL DEPENDENCE

Psychological Dependence is more a state of mind and will probably cause the least of your problems in quitting or staying off of tobacco products.

Think of Psychological dependence as a child's security blanket. You may have a real fear of giving up tobacco because you *think* you can't get along without tobacco. Just as a child has a fear of going out without its security blanket or going to bed without its teddy bear. This is more a lack of confidence or fear of failure. You will get over this aspect of your need for tobacco about as quickly as you'll get past your tobacco withdrawal symptoms ... in a matter of a few days. Psychological dependence is more likely to show itself as an anxiety over not having a pack of cigarettes where you can get to them easily as being deprived of your smoking. It is something like an angina patient who has an attack because he realizes he doesn't have his nitro glycerin tablets with him. Just having them in his pocket where he knows he can get at them if he needs them is enough to hold off many attacks. That is what psychological dependence means.

Confidence is what is necessary to get past psychological dependence.

HABITUATION...

Habituation or habit is your toughest obstacle. This program (QSN) will do all possible to help you get through the habit systems you have built up around your smoking through the years.

Habituation involves all the personal *"triggers"* developed over your entire smoking life that say to you, "You need a nicotine fix right now!" Understanding these triggers and being forewarned about them... becoming aware of them... recognizing them ... and thus being able to avoid them... is your best key to successfully remaining a non-smoker. QSN will spend most of its energies helping you to become aware of and avoid your smoking triggers.

All this addiction, psychological dependence, and especially habituation mean kicking the smoking habit is not easy, but it is possible.

Since it is nicotine that you are addicted to, we do not believe in using smokeless cigarettes, nicotine gum, nicotine tablets or other chemical crutches. All they do is keep your addiction and habit system alive. To be free of your addiction means to *stay away from nicotine in all forms and at all times!*

It is important to realize that over 70 to 90 million smokers have quit their habit and so can you. Many of those millions of ex-smokers were two, three and four packs a day smokers. They were just as addicted as you. They were just as scared as you are to make their commitment to quit. Their craving for their next smoke was just as strong as yours. They took as much pleasure from smoking as you did. They too decided enough was enough. Something finally motivated them enough to quit and that motivation helped them to succeed.

You too will succeed.

QSN will do everything it can to help you and support you in your efforts. It will be easier than you think because you won't be alone in your efforts to quit smoking forever. QSN is with you all the way until you know you're a non-smoker forever!

MOTIVATION

Motivation is the key to success in anything we achieve. Motivation in your effort to quit smoking must be stronger than your desire to once again take up smoking. Let's examine some of the motives to keep you from ever smoking again.

FACTS ABOUT
SMOKING AND HEALTH

You've probably heard all the facts about smoking and health before. But now there's a difference. Now *you're a non-smoker.* Now you may find it easier to accept the facts regarding the dangers of smoking. When you were a smoker, denial was easier than acceptance of these facts. Now that you're a non-smoker let's review them one more time and really think about them for a change.

Actually, the dangers to your health are probably not your strongest motivations to quit tobacco. It has been too easy for you to think or say, "It won't make much difference if I quit next month or next year!" Sound familiar? Well it does make a difference. Tomorrow ... next week ... next month ... next year will never come. You'll always put it off for another period of time. The only way to be sure you'll quit is to QUIT SMOKING NOW! Not tomorrow, not next week, not next month ... NOT

EVEN AFTER YOUR NEXT CIGARETTE ... It has to be NOW!

That's why *you are no longer a smoker.*

You have already quit! You did it NOW! You're committed! You've made your investment and now you are a non-smoker! Say that a few times to yourself, to see how it feels. "I'm a non-smoker!" Then say it to yourself if you're ever tempted to pick up another cigarette, for that smoke would be an end to that important personal commitment and make that investment worthless!

Yes, your smoking, up to now, has injured your health with every single cigarette you smoked. **Each and every cigarette hurt you!** Each one did serious damage to your health!

Quitting will help you regain good health. And yes, the earlier you quit, the more good health you will regain. It does make a very big difference when you quit. NOW! is the best time to quit!

WHAT DOES SMOKING DO TO SMOKERS?

Despite the denials of the Tobacco Institute, smoking is a serious hazard to human health and life. Up to 500,000 Americans die each year as a direct result of their smoking habit. Let me repeat that ...

A HALF-MILLION AMERICANS DIE EACH TWELVE MONTHS BECAUSE THEY USE TOBACCO IN ONE FORM OR ANOTHER!

That's in the U.S. alone; the world over it's far more.

It doesn't matter if you smoke cigarettes, cigars or a pipe, tobacco **eventually it will kill you if you return to it!**

Smokeless tobacco kills too. Chewing tobacco, snuff, tobacco in any form is poison to human tissue ... and poison kills!

The tobacco industry is the only industry I know of that shamelessly kills off up to 500,000 of its best customers each year in America alone. More amazing is that its customers don't seem to mind. They just keep on supporting the industry that's killing them. That's worse than suicide; it's like putting out a contract to kill on yourself!

Yes, tobacco kills tobacco users ... let us count the ways:

1. *Smokers die younger than non-smokers*. The fact is that the death rate of smokers **at all ages** is higher than for non-smokers. And that accelerated death rate climbs significantly in direct proportion to the number of cigarettes smoked, the number of years of smoking and how early an age the smoker began the habit. This means that smokers in their twenties have a higher death rate than non-smokers in their twenties. The same is true in the thirties, forties, fifties. The death rate for smokers accelerates at a much more rapid rate as each decade passes.

2. *A little smoke is deadly too*. Men who smoke less than a half a package of cigarettes a day have a death rate 60% higher than non-smokers. A one to two pack a day smoker has a 90% higher death rate than a non-smoking peer. Two or more packs a day smokers have a death rate 120% higher than non-smokers in their same age groups.

3. *This translates into over 1,300 unnecessary deaths each and every day of the year* in the United States alone. That is like five jumbo jets with over 250 passengers crashing every day and killing everyone aboard. This is more deaths each year than the total of all alcohol related deaths, drug related deaths, accidental deaths, murders, suicides, and deaths caused in war in any one year added together. Think about that! Let me repeat it because it is an outrageous fact:

More Americans die each year from the effects of tobacco use than the total of all alcohol related deaths ... added to all drug related deaths ... added to all accidental deaths ... added to all murders ... added to all suicides ... added to all deaths caused by war in any one year!

What kind of a value system allows such an industry to continue? What kind of mentality keeps people supporting and defending such an industry? Why aren't we as outraged at the tobacco industry as we are about other environmental issues? *Tobacco smoke is the greatest environmental hazard in the entire world!*

4. Smoking is the major risk factor in heart attacks. Heart attack is the major killer disease among Americans. The American Heart Association estimates that 25% of all fatal heart attacks are caused by smoking. That means *170,000 heart attack deaths per year* in the United States *are caused by smoking!*

5. Lung cancer is only the second most frequent cause of death among smokers, killing 130,000 Americans yearly. To add emphasis to this fact, *lung cancer is relatively rare among non-smokers* ... virtually non-existent ... unless that non-smoker lives or works with heavy smokers. The incidence of lung cancer increases directly with the quantity smoked.

6. Smokers die of emphysema at a much higher rate than non-smokers. Smokers suffer a much higher rate of bronchitis, pneumonia, upper airway infections, allergies, colds, flues, sinus infections and other lingering respiratory illnesses compared to non-smokers. These diseases can not only cause lingering deaths, but can cripple a person to the point where he or she cannot care for him or herself, be productive or enjoy even the simplest of life's pleasures. *The death toll from chronic obstructive lung disease is about 50,000 Americans per year.*

7. Smokers have about five times the normal risk of dying from mouth cancer. Smokers suffer almost ten times the risk of dying from cancer of the larynx. Smokers also have a far higher incidence of dying of cancers of the urinary bladder, pancreas, breasts and almost every other part of the body.
Now aren't you glad you are a non-smoker

8. If you are pregnant and smoke, your chance of having a miscarriage, a stillbirth, a premature baby, a sick baby or a baby with birth defects is significantly higher. A recent study has shown that 70% of all Sudden Infant Death Syndrome (SIDS) tragedies occur in cases where the mother smoked during her pregnancy and in a high incidence of the remaining 30% the mothers were exposed to smoking by spouses, co-workers or other acquaintances.

9. Smoking increases your blood pressure dangerously. High blood pressure is a major cause of brain hemorrhage, stroke, kidney disease, heart disease and other potentially crippling or lethal diseases.

10. If you are a woman on birth control pills and smoke, you have a much higher risk of suffering heart attack, stroke and crippling or fatal blood clots ... all at a relatively young age!

11. Smoking aggravates and increases the incidence and severity of ulcers, diabetes, hypertension, angina,

headaches, migraines, epilepsy, allergies, renal diseases, colon cancer, irritable bowel syndrome, gum diseases, dental problems and many other health problems. It is estimated that *up to 50% of all hospitalizations in the United States are tobacco related.*

Think about how much smokers are costing *you* a non-smoker in added medical insurance costs. When a smoker gets sick, smoking may dramatically reduce the beneficial effects of prescription medications or the accuracy of medical tests. Not only do smokers use hospital facilities more than non-smokers, their hospital stays are longer and require high-tech facilities which spiral the cost of medical care, i.e.; cardiac care, intensive care, by-pass surgery, cardioversion, heart pump, emergency room resuscitation, long term hospitalization, oxygen therapy, lung surgery, long term nursing care, etc., etc., etc. We non-smokers are subsidizing the high cost of smokers' medical care through high insurance premiums.

The list goes on and on and on.... Add them all together and the deaths from tobacco use soars to half a million Americans snuffed out each year. Think what it must come to the world over. The tobacco industry is a death industry. It should, it must be shut down.

12. Smoking causes or aggravates ED or erectile dysfunction. If you have erectile dysfunction due to hypertension, diabetes, medications, circulatory problems and smoke the tobacco use is probably aggravating or potentiating the problem to the point that quitting smoking may resolve the problem. If there is no other physical problem causing ED, tobacco use is the probable cause of ED. Quitting can and probably will reverse the problem. The same goes for women smokers; tobacco use can reduce sexual response for the same reasons and causes as for ED in men.

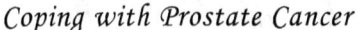
Coping with Prostate Cancer

IF NOT FOR YOU, THEN BE CONSIDERATE OF OTHERS!

A more tragic statistic than the fact that smoking kills a half million smokers per year, is the tragic fact that ... *side stream smoke kills up to 50,000 non-smokers each year!* If you smoked in the presence of others who are non-smokers, you contributed to the deaths of up to 50,000 innocent people who have made the choice not to smoke.

It is this danger to non-smokers that is causing all the strife between smokers and non-smokers everywhere. If a smoker wants to risk his or her life and health by smoking, he or she have that right ... but *smokers do not have the right to impose the same or worse danger on people who do not want to breathe side stream smoke.* Side stream smoke is not just an unpleasant nuisance.

Side stream smoke is the smoke that comes off of the lit end of a cigarette, cigar or pipe, polluting the air all around the smoker. It is a lethal air pollutant to all who are forced to inhale it. Most susceptible to these lethal gasses and chemicals are unborn fetuses, infants and children and the elderly.

Side stream smoke is far more deadly and poisonous than the mainstream smoke that the smoker inhales! How is this possible? When a cigarette, cigar or pipe is smoldering, the lit portion is a gray color. Its temperature is only around 250 degrees. The smoke pollution coming off its lit end and filling the air around it is cool and contains thousands of lethal chemical components. When the smoker draws on the cigarette, cigar or pipe the rush of air passing through the lit end suddenly brings it to life with a hot red glow and the temperature jumps up to over 1,000 to 1,200 degrees. Burning is far more efficient at 1,000 degrees than at 250 degrees. At the higher temperatures many of the lethal chemical parts are burned up so there are less of them in the smoke coming off the burning tobacco. Therefore, side stream smoke has up to 10 times more tar, 10 times more carbon monoxide, 50 times more benzenes, in fact many, many more times all of the thousands of poisonous chemical substances that have been analyzed out of tobacco smoke.

Knowingly smoking in the presence of children, born or unborn, is a form of child abuse ... **a *SILENT CHILD ABUSE!*** The child abuse caused by smoking in the presence of children is very real and far reaching. It abuses the child by doing both physical and mental damage which is too often irreversible. Volumes of evidence is now available showing side stream smoke is a tremendous hazard to our health ... and a far greater hazard to children whose bodies are growing, developing, whose cells and organ systems require a greater supply of fresh clean oxygen to develop to their maximum potential. Deterrents to this development in these maximum growth stages of life can never be made up in the future. If you, as a parent or grandparent, expose your children to side stream smoke, you are perpetrating a child abuse as surely as if you were overtly beating or otherwise harming the child. As a non-smoker, do not take your children into areas where they can be exposed to the smoke of others ... or you are also perpetrating an abuse.

Side stream smoke is devastating to children!

Again, side stream smoke kills up to 50,000 non-smokers each year! Let's examine some facts:

1. If you expose your non-smoking spouse to your side stream smoke, you increase his/her chances of developing lung cancer by over 90%. Yale University School of Medicine reported that non-smoking women whose husbands smoked more than 20 cigarettes a day are more than twice as likely to die of lung cancer as the wives of non-smokers. There are no figures for children yet, but the effect on them is probably far greater. One study showed that 5,000 non-smoking women die each year of lung cancer caused by exposure to heavy side stream smoke exposure from their spouses.

2. The Environmental Protection Agency (EPA) of the U.S. Government has stated, "Side stream smoke is deadlier than the primary smoke inhaled by the smoker!' Over two-thirds of the smoke from a cigarette goes into the air when a smoker inhales. When the cigarette smolders, all of the smoke goes into the surrounding air. The average cigarette burns from twelve to fourteen minutes. Only two minutes of that time is it being drawn on by the smoker. This means that the cigarette shoulders from ten to twelve minutes spewing well over 80% of its smoke pollution into the air that non-smokers have to breathe. Remember, the side stream smoke carries a measurably higher concentration of cancer-causing compounds than mainstream smoke actively inhaled by the smoker. Studies show conclusively that side stream smoke contains up to ten times more carbon-monoxide, up to ten times more tars, 50 times more ammonia, more cyanide and more benzene ... more of all the thousands of known poisonous chemicals in tobacco smoke. *And realize that the smoker not only gets the mainstream smoke but the side stream smoke as well!*

3. Carbon monoxide blood levels of a non-smoker doubles when exposed to a smoker, *even in a well ventilated room.* In fact, one smoker in a well ventilated room will raise the carbon monoxide levels to over double the maximum levels allowed for industrial workers by the federal government. Just think what it is like in a smoke filled work place where non-smokers have to spend eight hours a day.

4. It takes several hours for the blood levels of carbon monoxide in a child's, as well as an adult's, system to return to normal after being exposed to the side stream smoke of just <u>one cigarette</u>. If in that time, there is exposure to additional cigarettes, the levels continue to rise. A child who is exposed to the continuous smoking of a parent, relative or stranger, may never clear the excess carbon monoxide or cancer causing chemicals from its small body.

5. The lungs of children exposed to side stream smoke *do not grow as rapidly as those whose parents do not smoke.* Thus, children who are constantly exposed to smoke cannot get as much of the necessary oxygen into their systems to give them their full developmental potential.

6. Children whose parents smoke or who are taken into smoking areas regularly face increased risk of such breathing disorders as allergies, emphysema and bronchitis according to the *"New England Journal Of Medicine."*

7. An adult non-smoker in a smoke-filled room for one hour will inhale as much cancer-causing material as a smoker would after inhaling up to 30 cigarettes, according to a paper presented at a Joint American-Canadian Chemical Society conference.

8. Smoking is harmful to a developing fetus in a pregnant mother. *No pregnant woman should smoke.* A non-smoking pregnant woman should *never* allow herself to *be exposed to the smoke of her spouse or others.*

9. A recent study found a possible link between Sudden Infant Death Syndrome (SIDS) or Crib Death and smoking. Mothers of the infants who died of this tragic event either smoked or were exposed to a high concentration of side stream smoke in an overwhelming percentage of the cases.

10. The EPA states that over 5,000 non-smoking

Americans will die this year of *lung cancer* because they inhaled side stream smoke. This says nothing of the chronic lung disease, hypertension, heart disease and other ailments and terminal diseases caused by smoking that these innocent people and children are being exposed. *Up to forty-five thousand more non-smokers may have their lives shortened by these other smoke caused diseases.*

11. The EPA states that, **"Cigarette smoke is the most dangerous airborne pollutant** because it contains radioactive particles that can cause cancer."

12. Tobacco smoke is over 90 times more lethal than the dangers of Asbestos. Asbestos causes about 3,000 deaths a year *world wide.* Why don't we make as big a fuss over the deaths caused by the tobacco industry?

The above listed are facts which you can accept, or like the Tobacco Industry, pooh pooh. If you want to continue to court death and illness, that's your business, *but when you do your smoking in the presence of others who are non-smokers, it becomes the serious business of others.* **You have every right to destroy yourself, but you have no right to harm others while doing it, nor incur additional health care expense on them.**

For further fact on the dangers of side stream smoke we refer you to the U.S. Surgeon General's 1986 Report on Smoking and Health.

Hopefully, now that ***you are a non-smoker,*** you will speak up, when in the presence of a smoker. Speak up for yourself when you are *assaulted* by an inconsiderate smoker. And above all, speak up for defenseless infants and children who are exposed to smoke by a thoughtless parent, grandparent or other guardian. Speak up for a child who is constantly being subjected to side stream smoke by a thoughtless or non-caring parent or grandparent who will insist on taking his or her own pleasure in spite of the hazard it presents tot he child. This is nothing less than a **SILENT CHILD ABUSE.**

REASONS TO QUIT SMOKING OTHER THAN HEALTH

There are other reasons to quit smoking beside health factors. If your own health and the health of your loved ones isn't enough to turn you off of smoking forever, consider the *social reasons to quit.*

It is ironic that most of us started smoking for social reasons. Our peers did it and so we did it to be part of the gang. Peer pressure is the major reason most smoke; that or seeing our parents or grandparents do it. We find that peer pressure is one of the strongest reasons for quitting the smoking habit. Finally, popular opinion has turned against the smoker. Smoking is no longer "in." It has become an anti-social habit. Smokers are in a minority in the United States today. Depending on what part of the country you are in, what economic level you are part of and what your educational level is the percentage of smokers ranges from less than 20% to 35%. In any situation, non-smokers far outnumber smokers. The higher the economic and educational level of your peers, the lower the percentage of smokers you'll encounter.

What social factors make a smoker a less desirable companion?

IF YOU SMOKE,
YOU SMELL!

Most smokers can no longer detect the acrid odor on themselves or other smokers. If you want to know how you smell to those non-smokers around you, stick your nose deep into a dirty ashtray full of old cigarette or cigar butts and inhale deeply through your nose. That's how others smell you and at a distance of several feet. When a smoker enters a smoke free room, all the non-smokers in that room know a smoker has just entered, even if he or she isn't smoking at the time.

Your odor precedes you when you smoke.
Your breath smells of stale tobacco.
Your skin smells of stale tobacco
Your hair smells of stale tobacco
Your clothes reek of stale tobacco.

Now that you're a non-smoker take a long shower and shampoo and get your clothes thoroughly cleaned.

You'll notice people will be more comfortable around you. Also avoid others who smoke, because if you're around them very much you'll pick up their smoke odor from the side stream smoke.

After you've been a non-smoker for a few days your sense of smell will gradually return. You'll slowly begin to recognize the odor in your car, your home, in your clothes closet, in your dresser drawers, and you'll especially recognize it on other smokers. That, my friend, is what you've smelled like for as long as you've smoked.

While we're on the subject, let's dispel a myth about fragrances. Let's discuss pipe smokers a moment. It seems every pipe smoker thinks his pipe smells wonderful. That's because pipe smokers can't smell their own smoke. So they go out of their way to get the most aromatic tobacco they can buy. They think they're adding to the pleasure of others. Well that isn't the way it works. To non-smokers and other smokers, there are few odors more offensive than the pungent smell of aromatic pipe tobacco. Most people will agree that pipe smoke is even more disagreeable than cigar smoke. There is a reason why many places that allow smoking will not allow cigar or pipe smoking.

Burning tobacco simply stinks!

IF YOU SMOKE YOU MAKE A POOR IMPRESSION!

When you smoke around non-smokers who don't know you, their first impression is that you are inconsiderate of others, that you have poor judgment, that. you're of weak character and most of all, that you're a fool! Maybe those non-smokers who do know you think many of the same things. It's hard to respect a person who smokes in face of all the reasons not to smoke.

Smokers are indeed fools! Most are indeed inconsiderate of others! Smokers do indeed demonstrate poor judgment! And anyone who has quit the habit and those who never fell prey to it are bound to question the character of one who insists he or she "Just can't quit!"

Now that you have quit ... stay quit!

IF YOU SMOKE YOU'RE HURTING YOUR BUSINESS!

You probably can't begin to imagine how much business you've lost, sales you haven't closed or overhead you're causing by smoking. It's one thing smokers tend to deny. **Well, Open Your Eyes Already!!!**

You alienate non-smoking clientele when you smoke. Remember, about 75% of the general population does not smoke. They don't like to be near you because you have an unpleasant odor. If you smoke in your place of business, they do not like to enter. Non-smokers want to breathe clean air. Let us repeat, 75% of your potential clientele are non-smokers, (unless you own a tobacco store). If you allow smoking in your store, your merchandise reeks of tobacco. Non-smokers do not want to purchase items that smell of tobacco from sales people who also reek of tobacco from a store filled with air that smells of stale tobacco.

You increase overhead dramatically when you smoke in the work place. Government figures bear out the fact that each smoker costs his or her employer over $4,500 more each year than a non-smoker. This is due to increased insurance premiums, decreased production, lost time from work, increased cost of building and equipment maintenance and other increased overhead costs directly related to smoking. Companies which do not employ smokers can often save 25% to 35% on health, fire and life insurance premiums. At today's insurance costs that, in itself, is a tremendous savings in business overhead.

Smokers take two to four times as much sick leave as non-smokers in a non-smoking work place. In a work place that does force non-smokers to work in side stream smoke, the non-smokers also have a much higher incidence of absenteeism.

When you consider the wages paid during such loss of production that is indeed a heavy expense for employers to subsidize. Furthermore, studies show that maintenance costs can be cut by 50% when smoking is eliminated from the work place. Electronic equipment requires far less repair and cleaning. Interiors do not have to be cleaned as often. Furniture does not require cleaning, refinishing or replacement as often because of burns. Windows do not have to be washed as often. Carpeting does not require replacement or patching as often when smokers are kept out. **Remember, over 50% of all fire losses in this country are caused by careless smoking!**

These are the reasons why more and more companies are establishing a policy of hiring only non-smokers. Now, more and more companies are paying for their employees' participation in smoking cessation programs. Some are giving smokers the ultimatum, "Stop smoking ... or find a new job!"

One of the biggest employee problems employers have to face today is the dissention between smokers and their non-smoking fellow workers. It leaves employers one of two choices; go to the expense of putting in separate smoking areas with independent ventilation systems, or get rid of smokers. A word to the wise..

IF YOU SMOKE YOU'RE EXPENDABLE, NON-PROMOTABLE AND UNRELIABLE

Again, smokers have a significantly higher absenteeism than non-smokers. The higher incidence of upper respiratory infections, flu and other illnesses is responsible for more sick days. And non-smokers who are forced to breathe side stream smoke eight hours a day are made to suffer more allergies, colds, flu and upper respiratory problems. So more and more employers find the easiest and most cost effective solution is to get rid of smoking employees.

Last but not least, more and more often, smoking prevents you from getting into the board room. For many of the above reasons, smoking prevents you from advancements. All things equal, it will usually be the non-smoker who gets the advancement up the ladder. If you recall, statistics show overwhelmingly that the higher the economic and education level of individuals, the less likely they are to smoke. Look around you at the executives and top echelons in your organization. You'll discover a very small percentage of them smoke. Peek into the executive board rooms. There is seldom smoking there. Very few still allow ashtrays in. *The writing is on the wall....*

SMOKING COSTS YOU
MORE THAN JUST MONEY!!

If a pack of cigarettes costs $3.50 and the average smoker goes through two packs a day that totals: $2,555 per year or $212 per month.

The average worker works 2080 hours a year. If you quit smoking, it'd be like giving yourself a $1.22/hour raise *(in post-tax dollars, so it's more like a $1.75/hour raise)*! How often does that happen in this economy - now that were all looking down the barrel of a recession*. How likely is it that your employer is just going to decide to give you a raise that big for making a wise decision? They won't - **but you can**!

*If you'd like to find out how quitting smoking can help you become recession proof by using that money in a more intelligent way, get the book: "Secrets to Creating Passive Income" by EJ Thornton and John Clark Craig, *ISBN: 0980194199.*

That's just the cost of cigarettes, what about the health-care savings? What about the house cleaning savings? What about the cost of all the smoking-accessories - you're saving there too?

WHAT ARE YOUR REASONS FOR QUITTING?

QSN has given you a few of the good reasons to quit smoking now! **We have yet to find any *good* reasons for continuing the habit!**

There are many more reasons for quitting.

What are your personal reasons? Make a list of them. Your reasons are the most important ones. They are your beat motivation. Put down as many of them as you can after our listing and review them daily:

1. My health.
2. The health of my family and friends.
3. My job and professional goals.
4. Opinions of others.
5. Economics.
6. I'm sick of being badgered by non-smokers.
7. My family and friends are worried about my health.
8. I know I've got to do it sooner or later ... NOW! is the time.
9. I'm tired of being a victim and slave to the tobacco industry.
10. Smoking has a bad affect on my love and sex life.
11. I'm setting a horrible example for my kids.
12. I do not want to develop erectile dysfunction (ED) or have my sexual response diminished.

13...

14...

15...

16...

17...

18...

19...

20...

MAKE IT AS EASY AS POSSIBLE FOR YOURSELF!

There are a number of tricks to help you keep from ever smoking again.

Here are a few:

1. Get rid of all your smoking paraphernalia:
    Cigarettes
    Cigars
    Pipes
    Humidors
    Pipe stands
    Lighters
    Ashtrays
    Pipe cleaners and gadgets

2. Tell others that you have quit smoking and gain their support.

3. Take it one day at a time. Just make sure you don't let temptation get the best of you today. Tomorrow will take care of itself. Each day becomes easier than the last, so if you can make it through today, tomorrow will be easier. After the first two days, *just 48 hours,* it becomes a lot easier. It takes about that long for the physical addiction craving to wear off.

4. Remember, it may take 48 hours for the addiction cravings to wear off, but it only takes *one cigarette* to get you hooked again!

5. Avoid other smokers while they are smoking. First of all, their side stream smoke will injure your health and retard your

recovery from your own smoking. Second, their habit may add to your temptation in the first weeks of your new lifestyle. Just excuse yourself from them politely while they have their smoke. If they are at all considerate, they will not smoke in your presence. **Remind them you are a non-smoker now!**

6. Try to get others you know to give up smoking along with you. It is easier to "kick-it" with a friend or a loved one.

7. Observe others who still smoke from a distance. Watch how they are slaves to their habit. In a few days, you'll be able to notice how they smell. Observe how non-smokers tend to avoid them while they are puffing away.

8. Every time you think about smoking, put the cost of a pack of cigarettes away in savings toward a trip or other luxury you'd like to have or perhaps a gift for someone you care for.

9. Carry sugarless chewing gum and chew it whenever the urge to smoke hits you. If you don't like chewing gum, carry some celery or carrot sticks with you. And don't worry about gaining weight because you stopped smoking. We'll take care of that in the next part of this program.

10. When you feel the urge for a brief smoke break, go to a non-smoking area and spend a few minutes visiting. Talk about your urge and give your friend a chance to help you get over it.

11. If you can, take a brisk walk after meals when the urge for a smoke is often strongest. Exercise is an excellent, healthy way to get over or avoid a smoking urge.*

* A great walking program is detailed in "The Second Half Begins at 50 by Othniel J. Seiden M.D. and Jane L. Billet, PhD. ISBN: 0-9801941-1-3

12. Spend as much of your spare time in places where smoking is forbidden over the next few weeks, i.e.; Museums,

movies, galleries, visiting non-smoking friends, etc.

13. By the same token, for the next few weeks avoid places where smoking is prevalent, i.e.; bars, pool halls, restaurants without non-smoking sections, etc.

14. Try to avoid alcohol for the next few days. Smoking and alcohol seem to go together and furthermore, alcohol can lower your resolve and you may need all the perseverance you can muster for the next few days.

15. Throw a non-smoker's party in a couple of weeks to celebrate your victory over a real bad habit. Send the invitations NOW! That will make you stick to your resolve.

16. Your thoughts and tips to help **you** keep from smoking. (Hint: list the people and places to avoid, some trigger foods, etc).

....

....

....

....

....

....

....

....

....

TRIGGERS TO SMOKERS!!!

There are some very common triggers that say to the smoker as well you the ex-smoker, "Now I'd like a smoke!" These are situations in which you find yourself that call to you for a smoke. Let's look at some of them, unmask them, make you well aware of them and show you how to respond to or avoid them.

These triggers are not part of your addiction to nicotine; they are part of the habit system you've developed regarding your past smoking. The solution to the problems they cause is to replace them with new habit systems ... healthier habit systems.

1. I miss a smoke after a good meal!
a. Leave the table after the meal and take a brisk walk for about 15 minutes. That's about the time you'd have spent with your smoke. Walking is very healthy, aerobic, and it will decrease the urge to smoke dramatically.
b. Get up from the table and brush your teeth.
c. Chew some sugarless gum.

2. I miss having a smoke when I get a work break!
a. Take a brisk walk, outside if possible.
b. Take your break with other non-smokers.
c. Drink some fruit juice, tomato juice, vegetable cocktail, sugar free soda, ice tea, water, etc. Drinking tends to reduce the urge to smoke as long as you avoid coffee, booze or other hot drinks which usually invite smokers to light up.

3. I get an urge to smoke when I have a cup of coffee!
a. Take your coffee break with other non-smokers.
b. Reduce the amount of or avoid coffee altogether for a few days.

c. Replace coffee with fruit juices, vegetable juices, sugarless gum or take a brief exercise break.

4. When I'm under pressure, I want to smoke!

a. Remember, tobacco does not help you to solve your problems, *it actually adds to them.*

b. When you have a problem, take the time to thoroughly analyze it, then get away from it for a short while by switching to some other subject. Taking a long walk or other form of exercise, or just sit and daydream. Walking, exercising or daydreaming lets your right brain take over, which is your creative side of the brain. Most great ideas and accomplishments come from right brain activity, almost as revelations.

5. When I watch television, I automatically get the urge for a smoke!

a. Reduce the amount of television you watch for the next week or two.

b. When you do watch T.V., watch with non-smokers.

c. Do not allow smoking in your home or have any smoking paraphernalia available.

d. Go to movies, plays, lectures, museums or other entertainments where smoking is not allowed, in place of T.V. watching for a few weeks.

6. When I see others smoking, I want to join in with them

a. Avoid smokers for the next two weeks. Spend more time with non-smokers. Let them know you have just quit. They will be very happy to help you and you'll probably make some new good friends. Remember, 85% of all smokers want to quit their habit. They will also be willing to help you if they are true friends. And if you're a true friend you'll help them to quit too.

7. Playing cards gives me the yen for a smoke!

a. Don't play cards for a while.

b. Play cards with non-smokers.

c. Make it table rules that there be no smoking in the room or home where you play. To make that easier to enforce, be willing to host the game. If the players don't go along with your table rules, find a new game. It is interesting that more and more casinos are making non-smoking rooms available. Las Vegas, is waking up!

8. When I'm alone or feeling lonely I want a smoke!

a. Now that you're a non-smoker you'll find it easier to make new friends. Spend more time with people; seek out new activities.

b. Take long walks or other forms of exercise.

c. Spend time in places where smoking is not allowed art galleries, museums, movie theaters, the library, join a health club or gym, etc.

9. When I talk on the phone, I get an urge to smoke!

a. Avoid the phone! Keep conversations short when you do have to call someone.

b. Use E-mail or text message which keep both of your hands busy.

10. When I have a conflict with someone, I feel like smoking!

a. Seek a rational solution to the conflict. Smoking does nothing to resolve a problem. Talk it out. If nothing seems to break the deadlock, break off for a while. Take a long walk. Change the subject. Give the right brain a chance to resolve the conflict.

b. Try to see the conflict from the other person's viewpoint then retry settling the argument. *Remember, smoking solves nothing!*

11. As soon as I sit down in a car, I want to smoke.

a. Remember, smoking in a car, even with the windows down is like riding in a gas chamber.

b. Try to take a non-smoker in the car with you.

c. If it's a short trip consider walking or biking.

d. If it's a long trip consider taking public transportation for a few weeks.

e. If it's a regular drive, like driving to work every day, consider car pooling with non-smokers.

f. Thoroughly clean the inside of your car and make it a strict non-smoking vehicle. Never let anyone smoke in your car. Never ride in someone else's car while he or she smokes. It's lethal!

12. I get the urge to smoke when I'm in a restaurant!

a. Only go to restaurants that offer a non-smoking section (or is completely smoke-free) and always insist on being seated as far away from the smokers as possible.

b. If your community does not have non-smoking laws for restaurants or public places, become an activist and work with other non-smokers to get such ordinances passed. It has worked in many cities, counties and states, pushed through by people just like you who are sick and tired of having to breathe other peoples' disgusting smoke.

13. I get the urge to smoke when I'm in a bar!

a. Stay out of bars for the next three to four weeks.

b. It's much cheaper to drink at home with non-smoking friends; but for the next four weeks try to avoid booze because it increases the desire to smoke.

I'M AFRAID THAT IF I QUIT SMOKING I'LL GAIN WEIGHT!

Most people *do not* gain significant weight when they quit smoking! There is some evidence that smoking may speed up ones metabolism a little, but it is not usually the act of quitting smoking that causes those who do gain to put on weight.

It is typically replacing the smoking habit with the snacking habit that causes this. Snacking, even at its very worst, is far healthier than smoking. **You would have to gain to about 75 pounds over your ideal weight* to put your health at the same risk as smoking.** The best thing you can possibly do is to quit smoking and join a health club. That will really improve your health. If you don't want to join a gym, then join a friend, your spouse, a neighbor, your kids or a group from work and exercise walk together. Chances are your weight will drop in spite of quitting smoking.

* To find out your ideal weight, look into the book "Heavy and Healthy" by Othniel J. Seiden and Jane L. Bilett, PhD. ISBN: 0-9779960-5-0

THE MYTH ABOUT EXCESSIVE WEIGHT GAIN WHEN YOU QUIT SMOKING!

Most ex-smokers do *not* replace their nicotine habit with excessive snacking. That's a myth the Tobacco Institute loves to see perpetuated. Many smokers, especially women are afraid to quit for fear of gaining too much weight. To make sure you don't fall into the snacking habit, let's give you some common sense tips on avoidance:

1. I'm afraid I'll nibble and snack all day in place of smoking!

a. Carry sugarless gum or mints to use in place of candy and other high caloric sweets.

b. Keep celery and carrot sticks available to munch.

c. Drink tea, tomato juice, vegetable juices, unsweetened fruit juices or bouillon in place of high caloric soft drinks and colas.

d. Other low caloric snacks that you should keep available are tomato wedges, green red or yellow pepper strips, fresh mushrooms, broccoli or cauliflower bits, radishes, turnip slices and cucumber slices.

2. I get an urge to eat when I'm under stress. Those were the times I used to smoke!

a. Find other stress reducing activities ... walking or other forms of exercise and hobbies.*

* A good list of easy, stress reducing, life enhancing hobbies is listed in: "The Second Half Begins at 50" by Othniel J. Seiden M.D. and Jane L Bilett, Ph.D. ISBN: 0-9801941-1-3

b. Practice defensive food shopping. Don't stock up on high calorie, high sugar content, high-fat foods. If they're not in your refrigerator or cupboards, you won't be able to snack on them. On the other hand, make healthy snack foods readily available. Among these are raw vegetables, fresh fruits, un-buttered popcorn, juices (unsweetened), bouillon, tea, coffee, diet drinks, sugarless gum and candies. Carbonated water is excellent to drink over the rocks or to mix with fruit juices as coolers and will lowering the fruit drink's caloric content even lower.

QUITTING SMOKING IS, IN FACT, NO EXCUSE TO GAIN WEIGHT!

WEIGHT GAIN IS NO EXCUSE FOR NOT QUITTING SMOKING!

GETTING BACK INTO SHAPE

Your past smoking has damaged your health! If you return to smoking at any time in the future, that damage will continue at an accelerating rate. If you never smoke again, your health status will improve considerably.

There are steps you can take to dramatically speed your health improvement. With some relatively simple changes in your lifestyle you can get yourself into the best physical condition you've ever been in; recover from much of the damage you've done to yourself and add productive, quality years to your life. *A LIFE-LONG SMOKER WILL LIVE ABOUT 18 YEARS LESS THAN HIS or HER NON-SMOKING PEERS.* That is a lot of life wasted.

By quitting now, you will save many of those 18 years for yourself and loved ones to enjoy. You've already done the most important thing ... quit smoking and avoiding other people's side stream smoke!

In addition, this simple program to get you back into shape will also prevent you from gaining weight because you stopped smoking. Follow this program and you'll be in the best shape you've ever known.

Since your smoking has done most of its damage to your cardiovascular and respiratory systems, this reshaping program is aimed mainly at restoring them back to their maximum potential health. But while reshaping these most important life systems, you will also be lowering your blood pressure, reducing your stress levels, diminishing your body fat ratio and building up and toning muscle tissue, improving your endurance, lowering your cholesterol and generally making yourself over into a healthy person. And the best part of all this is ... it's painless! You'll probably even enjoy it! Think of it ... something fun and enjoyable that's actually healthy for you!

YOUR *PAINLESS* EXERCISE PROGRAM

Now that you are no longer a smoker, you should continue to achieve the best physical and mental health within your potential. To accomplish this you need a good aerobic exercise program. The simplest, safest, most natural and best human aerobic exercise is walking. If you will work up to a one hour brisk walk daily, you will be getting the ideal workout ... better than swimming, jogging, cycling or any court sport.

If for some physical reason walking is out of the question for you, then find another exercise you can take part in vigorously. If, for example, you have severe arthritis, then consider swimming as your main activity. Just as it is never too late to quit smoking, it is never too late to start a vigorous exercise program.

GET RID OF YOUR OTHER BAD HABITS

Smokers have a higher incidence of other addictions than do the general public. If you have been addicted to tobacco, you have a greater potential to become addicted to other chemicals. You must face the fact that you have an "addictive potential." At least one in ten people in the general public is addicted to alcohol, prescription drugs, hard drugs or a combination of the above listed. Though less than a third of the general population now smokes, the addiction rate to other chemicals in that smaller population is about one in three. Let's reemphasize this fact, *"one in three smokers is addicted* to alcohol, prescription drugs such as tranquilizers, pain killers, cold remedies or sedatives, or, hard drugs like marijuana, cocaine, heroin, etc. Often the addiction is to more than one of the above!

If you find you are drinking more than "socially"... more than a drink or two daily ...drinking every day ... take a hard look at your "drinking habit!" If you have been on any prescription medication for more than two weeks, discuss it with your doctor. Make him explain the need for continued use of the prescription. If it is justified, by all means, follow his or her instructions to the letter. But you should know everything about anything you ingest into your body.

If you are using any over-the-counter medication for a prolonged period, discuss it with your pharmacist or physician. Find out the dangers of its prolonged use.

If you are using any illegal drug **GET HELP NOW!** It will not only kill you ... it will ruin whatever life you have left while you use it!

Again, if you are using alcohol, drugs or medications to excess, **GET HELP NOW!**

CREATE YOUR OWN
SUPPORT GROUP!

How does the support group help you?

It is easier to do anything when you have the support of others. We all like to be cheered along and rewarded for our successes. And when the going gets a little tough, the helping hand and encouragement from a friend can do wonders. That's what a support group is all about. QUIT SMOKING NOW! offers you continuing support, now or weeks, months, years from now, should you need it. Review this material frequently. It will strengthen your resolve. Let friends, family and loved ones help you. In a support group, you'll be helping others as well. That's important. When you help others who are trying to quit smoking, it's virtually impossible for you to backslide. If you are quitting on your own, without going through the QSN program classes, try to get others to do this with you; friends, family members, fellow workers. They will then make up your support group.

INTRODUCTION TO THE SUPPORT GROUP.

How do you keep from falling off the wagon? Get active in anti-smoking activities. It is difficult to fall off the wagon when you are trying to help others. Become a clean air activist. Help others "kick cold turkey." Consider becoming a QUIT SMOKING NOW! group leader. Become active in a QUIT SMOKING NOW! support group.

Remember ... THIS IS FOR LIFE!

Smoking is an addiction. You can never start again without getting hooked. Don't even try. Total avoidance is the only way to stay on the wagon. If you do try another smoke, you'll be as hooked as you were when you quit. You will have to go through the same steps you have just been through to kick the habit again. You'll have to quit cold turkey....

To help you avoid smoke at work, post the following memo to smokers.

Memo to smokers:

Please show courtesy and consideration to non-smokers so no one's rights have to be restricted. We are referring to the rights of smokers to smoke and the rights of non-smokers to breathe clean, healthy air. This is not just a matter of unpleasant odors in the air. Many of the 70% non-smokers are allergic to smoke. It causes severe burning of the eyes, sore throat, upper respiratory distress, headache, nausea, colds and flu! etc.

Strife between smokers and non-smokers can hopefully be averted with simple consideration.

1. Please, do not smoke at your own desk if it means a non-smoker near you will be forced to breathe your side stream smoke.

2. Please, do not smoke when walking through the building.

3. Please, do not smoke in the rest rooms.

4. Please, do not smoke at the copy machines or other public areas.

5. Please, do not smoke in areas where non-smokers have to work and share the air.

Understand, no one is trying to infringe on your right to smoke, but second hand or side stream smoke is extremely dangerous to the health of smokers and non-smokers. Non-smokers have the right to breathe clean air.

Thank you, from your non-smokers fellow workers.

THE SILENT CHILD ABUSE

Though some of the following is repetition, it's reemphasis for those of you who have children or grandchildren. It is vitally important that you understand it in relation to your kids or grandchildren or any other child you comes in contact with smokers be they you or anyone else!

Child abuse has gotten a lot of press in recent years, as well it should. It's a fortunate thing that media has brought this horrible problem out of the closet. Yet there is a form of child abuse even more far reaching than the recently publicized form and what's worse it is perpetrated by people who "*dearly love their children.*" Most perpetrators of this silent child abuse would be shocked to realize their guilt and how serious and far reaching the effects are.

The silent child abuse usually begins even before birth of the victim. Physicians are lax in warning against it even when they recognize its signs. This silent child abuse involves both first hand and side stream smoke.

As a physician Othniel, some time ago, decided to put his efforts into making life safer for those of us who want to avoid the carcinogens and lethal effects of smoke but are forced to inhale these poisons because of lack of consideration by smokers.

Most susceptible to these lethal gasses and chemicals are unborn fetuses, infants and children.

Tragically, smoking parents, grandparents, relatives, acquaintances and strangers are abusing them assaulting our young ... almost constantly. Knowingly or unknowingly smoking in the presence of children, born or unborn, is nothing short of ***CHILD ABUSE!***

Child abuse caused by smoking in the presence of children abuses the child by doing both physical and mental damage ... too often irreversible damage.

Let's take a closer look at the effects of what we call side stream smoke.

Side stream smoke is smoke we are exposed to when we breathe the air contaminated by smokers in our vicinity. Volumes of evidence are now available showing side stream smoke is a tremendous hazard to our health. **This is a far greater hazard to children whose bodies are growing, whose cells and organ systems require a greater supply of fresh clean oxygen to develop to maximum potential.** Retardation to development in these maximum growth stages can never be made up in the future. If you as a parent or grandparent exposing your children to side stream smoke, you are harming your child's health and future potential. If you are a non-smoker but still take your children into areas where they are exposed to the smoke of others, you are still harming them.

Side stream smoke is devastating to children. Let's take a look at some facts:

1. The Environmental Protection Agency (E.P.A.) of the U.S. Government has stated, "Side stream smoke is deadlier than the primary smoke inhaled by the smoker!" Over four-fifths of the smoke from the cigarette goes into the air around the smoker. The side stream smoke contains a measurable higher concentration of cancer-causing compounds than the mainstream or smoker-inhaled smoke. Studies show conclusively that side stream smoke contains seven times more carbon monoxide and tar and 50 times more ammonia than the smoker-inhaled mainstream smoke.

2. Carbon monoxide blood levels of non-smokers double when exposed to smokers even in well ventilated room. These numbers increase and are far more damaging to children whose

respiratory rates are higher than those of an adult. In fact, one smoker in a well ventilated room will raise the carbon monoxide levels to over double the maximum level allowed for industrial workers by the federal government.

3. It takes several hours for the blood levels of carbon monoxide in a child's, as well as an adult's, system to return to normal after being exposed to the side stream smoke of **just one cigarette**. If in that time he or she is exposed to additional smoke, the levels continue to rise. A child who is exposed to the continuous smoking of a parent, relative or strangers may never clear the excess carbon monoxide or 4,000 other harmful chemicals in tobacco smoke from his or her small body.

4. Yale University School of Medicine reports that non-smoking women whose husbands smoke more than 20 cigarettes a day are over 100% more likely to die of lung cancer than the wives of non-smokers. There are no figures for children yet but the harm is far greater.

5. The lungs of children exposed to side stream smoke do not grow as rapidly as those whose mothers do not smoke.

6. Children whose parents smoke or who are taken into smoking areas regularly face increased risk of such breathing disorders as allergies, emphysema and bronchitis, according to the *"New England Journal Of Medicine,"*

7. An adult non-smoker in a smoke filled room for one hour will inhale as much cancer-causing materials as a smoker would after inhaling up to 30 cigarettes according to a paper presented at a *Joint American-Canadian Chemical Society* conference.

8. Smoking is harmful to a developing fetus in a pregnant mother. No pregnant woman should smoke. A non-smoking

pregnant woman should never allow herself to be exposed to the smoke of her spouse or others. Side stream smoke may be even more hazardous to a pregnant woman than if she smoked herself.

9. Recent studies show that Sudden Infant Death Syndrome (SIDS) or Crib Death is related to smoking. 70% of the mothers of SIDS cases smoked during pregnancy. Of the 30% who didn't, a great majority were exposed to the side stream smoke of their husbands or others in their daily environment.

10. Up to 50,000 non-smoking Americans will have their lives shortened this year because they regularly inhaled side stream smoke. Over 5,000 will die of lung cancer alone. The rest will die of chronic lung disease, hypertension, heart disease and other ailments and terminal diseases caused by smoke to which these innocent people and children are being exposed.

11. The EPA states that **"cigarette smoke is the most dangerous airborne pollutant because it contains radioactive particles which cause cancer."** The lethal effects of side stream smoke has been estimated (EPA) at 90 times greater than Asbestos.

To the above facts, The American Tobacco Institute states, "...the side effects of second-hand smoke are 'negligible and quite small.'" William Awlward, spokesman for the Tobacco Institute said, "If you accept that the National Institute of Health study is (even) close to the truth, then you must also accept that (second-hand cigarette smoke) is not a health issue, but a nuisance issue." When 50,000 innocent people die this year due to inhaling someone else's smoke that is indeed quite a "nuisance!" Ask someone who has lost a loved one if it is "just a nuisance matter." Ask Othniel!

Smoking is not a moral issue but the industry's denial of responsibility for the deaths and ill health of millions of humans is a gross immorality.

These are facts which you can accept or like the Tobacco Industry 'pooh-pooh.' If you want to continue to court death and illness, that's your business; but when you do your smoking in the presence of others who are non-smokers, it becomes the serious business of those others. You have every right to destroy yourself but you have no right to harm others while doing it.

Hopefully adult non-smokers will speak up for themselves when assaulted by the lack of consideration by a smoker. But what about the child who is brought into a smoking area by parent, grandparent or other guardian? Or a child who is constantly being subjected to side stream smoke by a thoughtless or non-caring parent or grandparent who will continue to insist on taking his or her own pleasure in spite of the hazard it presents to the child? This is nothing less than a *Silent Child Abuse!*

What should be done to prevent this
SILENT CHILD ABUSE?

1. If you are a parent or grandparent ***Quit Smoking Now!*** Not only will this keep you from contaminating the air your child or grandchildren breathe, it will prevent you from setting a poor example. Children learn by emulating those they love and respect. Don't give them a deadly habit to copy.

2. If you've convinced yourself you can't quit then at least don't smoke in the presence of children. In fact, do not smoke in the space they will occupy for at least three hours before they arrive and then ventilate the space thoroughly. If ***they*** can smell it when they come in, you haven't clean it up enough.

3. If you really care for others around, you don't smoke in the presence of anyone who is not himself a smoker. Don't even ask if it's alright for you to smoke. They may say okay, but the side stream smoke will still be injuring them. Just ask them, **"Is it alright if I poison you?"**

4. Do not ever take a child into a smoking area of a restaurant. In the hour it takes you to eat that meal, the child may get the equivalent damage of smoking two packs of cigarettes.
   Would you offer any child two packs of cigarettes?

5. If you are pregnant, do not expose yourself ... or allow yourself to be exposed to cigarette smoke. If you smoke, quit! Quit now! If you live with a smoker make that smoker quit! and quit now! DO NOT ALLOW ANYONE TO SMOKE IN YOUR PRESENCE! Refuse to go into any public place that does not have a non-smoking area! Demand clean air for yourself and your unborn child!

6. If your spouse is a non-smoker have the decency never to smoke in your their presence. You love them, don't you?

7. If children live in your home or visit there frequently, never smoke in your home or let anyone else smoke there. Carcinogens have a way of hanging around in the air.

8. Do not go into buildings where smoking is prevalent.

9. Speak up when someone else's smoke is polluting the air you have to breathe. Be insistent if your child has to breathe it. Would you allow someone to serve you or your child a glass of dirty water? Dirty air is far more harmful.

10. Become active in movements to provide the community with clean air and a smoke-free environment.

11. Smokers are like the plague. Over the years smoking has killed far more people than the plague! Avoid them like you would avoid the plague!

12. MAKE SURE NO ONE CAN EVER ACCUSE YOU OF CHILD ABUSE... THE SILENT CHILD ABUSE...

###

QSN has put a great deal of emphasis on the elimination of tobacco from your life. It is a must. We've tried to give you every reason we can imagine for you to quit. As serious as the problems of alcohol and illicit drugs are, in this country tobacco kills many times more people each year than all the drugs and alcohol put together. Even if you add to them all deaths from murder, suicide, accidents and war, tobacco kills more!!! This does not diminish the seriousness of other addictions. If you have any addictions to any chemical substances get help to kick them now! Your life and perhaps the lives of your loved ones, depend on it!

DOCTORS TO THE WORLD
Mission Statement:

DOCTORS TO THE WORLD is a charitable, service organization qualified and recognized by the United States government with tax deductible status, 501 (C)(3), dedicated to aiding the underprivileged, here and abroad, with health science services, education, as well as economic and environmental improvement.

MEDICAL SERVICES of Doctors To The World bring volunteer medical personnel ... physicians, nurses, technical and support people ... into areas of vital need, in the United States or the world over in a maximum cost effective way.

EDUCATION services of DTTW includes an active speakers bureau making information available to schools, groups, industry and developing countries. DTTW brings volunteer educators, technical and skilled persons into underprivileged areas to help the people develop knowledge and talent to improve and maintain a better lifestyle.

DISPLACED PERSONS services of DTTW works with refugees in foreign lands, such as the Miskito Indians in Honduras as well as homeless street people in our own cities.

CLEAN INDOOR AIR COALITION (CIAC) is a branch of DTTW dedicated to educating people about the major indoor air pollutant injuring our health ... side stream tobacco smoke. Through CIAC, Doctors To The World sponsors QUIT SMOKING NOW!, a smoking cessation program available to the public, industry ... and offered to public schools and you at no cost.

You can help in the continuing efforts of Doctors To The World by by sending your tax deductible contributions to:

Doctors To The World
P.O. Box 37167
Denver, Colorado 80237

To you,
the new non-smoker...

CONGRATULATIONS!!!

Sincerely,
Othniel J. Seiden, M.D.
Jane L. Bilett, Ph.D.
EJ Thornton (Publisher)
Doctors To The World!!!

Please feel free to share this with
anyone who still smokes!

Keeping our indoor air clean!

More From Othniel

Health

5 HTP The Serotonin Connection:
*The Natural Supplement that helps
you be in control of your mind and body!*
ISBN: 1519148445
5-HTP and Depression Management:
Available in Kindle Only
5HTP and Memory Loss Management with:
Available in Kindle Only
5 HTP PMS and Menopause:
Available in Kindle Only
Coping with Arthritis:
ISBN: 151941353X
Coping with BPH:
*Benign Prostatic Hypertrophy
Male, over 45, you probably have it!*
Available in Kindle Only
Coping with Colorectal Cancer:
*Prevention and Cure of theSecond Leading
Cause of Cancer Deaths*
Available in Kindle Only
Coping with Fibromyalgia:
It's not in your head, it's a disease!
ISBN: 1519438311

Coping with Prostate Cancer:
Prevention and Cure
of Man's Most Common Cancer
ISBN: 1519438737

Heart of a Woman:
Prevetion and Cure of the #1 Killer in Women
ISBN: 1519441533

Heavy and Healthy:
Forget Your Weight and Get Fit!
ISBN: 1519495412

Quit Smoking Now!:
The Program to Help You
Quit Smoking Now and Forever!
ISBN: 1519495781

Sharpening the Aging Mind:
Methods, Tricks & Tips to
Keep Your Mind Super Sharp
ISBN: 1519496028

Sleep Disorders Management:
Available in Kindle Only

The Second half begins at 50:
Your Longevity Handbook
ISBN: 1519496389

Walk!:
Walk Your Way to Great Health & Long Life
Available in Kindle Only

Weight & Appetite Management:
Available in Kindle Only

Relationships:

Adultery Case Histories:
> *Why People Cheat on Their Partners*
> **Available in Kindle Only**

Communing with the Dead:
> *Death Needn't Part You*
> ISBN: 1519190085

Foreplay:
> *The True Focus of Great Sex*
> ISBN: 1519440979

Sex in the Golden Years:
> *The Best Sex Ever, Stay Sexually Active for Life*
> ISBN: 1519495927

The Big O:
> *Male & Female Multiple Orgasms*
> ISBN: 1519496109

The Hospice Experience:
> *Making Your Most Important Final Decision*
> ISBN: 1519496281

When Your Spouse Dies:
> *A widow's & widower's handbook*
> ISBN: 151949646X

Jewish Fiction

Padre Pio:
> *The Capuchin – the life of Padre Pio -*
> *St. Pio of Pietrelcina*
> *Sex, Horror & Violence vs. Unyielding Faith!*
> ISBN: 1519495684

Seed of Avraham:
> *A 4000 Year History of the Jewish Family...*
> > **ISBN: 1519495811**

Shtetl:
> > *The Story of a Life No More...*
> > *As told from the hereafter*
> > > **ISBN: 1519496036**

The Cartographer:
> > *1492*
> > > **ISBN: 151949615X**

The Condemned Voyage:
> > *The S.S. St. Louis - 1939*
> > > **Available in Kindle Only**

The Crusades:
> *The Jewish World of the 12th Century*
> > **Available in Kindle Only**

The Death of Berlin:
> *A Story of Hollocaust Survival and Revenge*
> > **Available in Kindle Only**

The Remnant:
> *The Jewish Resistance in WWII*
> > **ISBN: 1519496346**

The Uprising of Babi Yar:
> > *The Syrets Deathcamp*
> > > **Available in Kindle Only**

Miscellaneous

Guaranteed Routes to Success for Writers:
> *A Road Map Through Today's*
> *Dramatic Changes in Publishing*
> > **Available in Kindle Only**

Joy of Volunteering:
Working and Surviving in Developing Countries
ISBN: 1519495587

So You Want to Write a Book:
ISBN: 1519496079

If you found

Coping with Prostate Cancer

helpful and useful

Please leave a review on Amazon.com

Also available in Kindle